Current Clinical Strategies

Gynecology and Obstetrics

2002 Edition

With ACOG Guidelines

Paul D. Chan, M.D.

Christopher R. Winkle, M.D.

Current Clinical Strategies Publishing

www.ccspublishing.com/ccs

Digital Book and Updates

Purchasers of this book can download the digital book and updates of this book via the internet at www.ccspublishing.com/ccs

Current Clinical Strategies Publishing
27071 Cabot Road
Laguna Hills, California 92653

Phone: 800-331-8227
Fax: 800-965-9420
Internet: www.ccspublishing.com/ccs
E-mail: info@ccspublishing.com

Printed in USA   ISBN 1929622-04-X

Contents

Surgical Documentation for Gynecology

Gynecologic Surgical History

Identifying Data. Age, gravida (number of pregnancies), para (number of deliveries).

Chief Compliant. Reason given by patient for seeking surgical care.

History of Present Illness (HPI). Describe the course of the patient's illness, including when it began, character of the symptoms; pain onset (gradual or rapid), character of pain (constant, intermittent, cramping, radiating); other factors associated with pain (urination, eating, strenuous activities); aggravating or relieving factors. Other related diseases; past diagnostic testing.

Obstetrical History. Past pregnancies, durations and outcomes, preterm deliveries, operative deliveries.

Gynecologic History: Last menstrual period, length of regular cycle.

Past Medical History (PMH). Past medical problems, previous surgeries, hospitalizations, diabetes, hypertension, asthma, heart disease.

Medications. Cardiac medications, oral contraceptives, estrogen.

Allergies. Penicillin, codeine.

Family History. Medical problems in relatives.

Social History. Alcohol, smoking, drug usage, occupation.

Review of Systems (ROS):

    General: Fever, fatigue, night sweats.

    HEENT: Headaches, masses, dizziness.

    Respiratory: Cough, sputum, dyspnea.

    Cardiovascular: Chest pain, extremity edema.

    Gastrointestinal: Vomiting, abdominal pain, melena (black tarry stools), hematochezia (bright red blood per rectum).

    Genitourinary: Dysuria, hematuria, discharge.

    Skin: Easy bruising, bleeding tendencies.

Gynecologic Physical Examination

General:

Vital Signs: Temperature, respirations, heart rate, blood pressure.

Eyes: Pupils equally round and react to light and accommodation (PERRLA); extraocular movements intact (EOMI).

Neck: Jugular venous distention (JVD), thyromegaly, masses, lymphadenopathy.

Chest: Equal expansion, rales, breath sounds.

Heart: Regular rate and rhythm (RRR), first and second heart sounds, murmurs.

Breast: Skin retractions, masses (mobile, fixed), erythema, axillary or supraclavicular node enlargement.

Abdomen: Scars, bowel sounds, masses, hepatosplenomegaly, guarding, rebound, costovertebral angle tenderness, hernias.

Genitourinary: Urethral discharge, uterus, adnexa, ovaries, cervix.

Extremities: Cyanosis, clubbing, edema.

Neurological: Mental status, strength, tendon reflexes, sensory testing.

Laboratory Evaluation: Electrolytes, glucose, liver function tests, INR/PTT, CBC with differential; X-rays, ECG (if >35 yrs or cardiovascular disease), urinalysis.

Assessment and Plan: Assign a number to each problem. Discuss each problem, and describe surgical plans for each numbered problem, including preoperative testing, laboratory studies, medications, and antibiotics.

Preoperative Note

Preoperative Diagnosis:
Procedure Planned:
Laboratory Data: Electrolytes, BUN, creatinine, CBC, liver function tests, INR/PTT, UA, EKG, chest X-ray; type and screen for blood or cross match.
Consent: Document explanation of risk and benefits of procedure to patient. Document explanation of alternatives to the procedure to the patient. Document patient's informed consent and understanding of the procedure.
Allergies:
Major Medical Problems:
Medications:

Brief Operative Note

Date of the Procedure:
Preoperative Diagnosis:
Postoperative Diagnosis:
Procedure:
Operative Findings:
Names of Surgeon and Assistant:
Anesthesia: General, spinal, or epidural.
Estimated Blood Loss (EBL):
Fluids and Blood Products Administered:
Urine output:
Specimens: Pathology specimens, cultures, blood samples.
Drains:

Operative Report

Identifying Data: Name of patient, medical record number; name of dictating physician, date of dictation.
Date of Procedure:
Preoperative Diagnosis:
Postoperative Diagnosis:
Procedure Performed:
Names of Surgeon and Assistants:
Type of Anesthesia Used:
Estimated Blood Loss (EBL):
Fluid and Blood Products Administered:
Specimens: Pathology, cultures, blood samples.
Drains and Tubes Placed:
Complications:
Indications for Surgery: Brief history of patient and indications for surgery.
Findings:
Description of Operation: Position of patient; skin prep and draping; location and type of incision; details of procedure from beginning to end including description of findings, both normal and abnormal, during surgery. Hemostatic and closure techniques; dressings applied. Needle and sponge counts as reported by operative nurse.
Disposition: The patient was taken to the recovery room in stable condition.
Copies: Send copies of report to surgeons.

Postoperative Orders

1. **Transfer** from recovery room to surgical ward when stable.
2. **Vital Signs:** q4h x 24h.
3. **Activity:** Bed rest; ambulate in 8 hours if tolerated. Incentive spirometer q1h while awake.
4. **Diet:** NPO x 8h, then sips of water. Advance to clear liquids, then to regular diet as tolerated.
5. **IV Fluids:** D5 ½ NS at 125 cc/h with KCL 20 mEq/L Foley to gravity.
6. **Medications:**
   Cefazolin (Ancef) 1 gm IVPB q8h x 3 doses.
   Meperidine (Demerol) 50-75 mg IM or IV q3-4h prn pain.
   Promethazine (Phenergan) 25-50 mg, IV q3-4h prn nausea **OR**
   Prochlorperazine (Compazine) 10 mg IV q3-6h prn nausea.
7. **Laboratory Evaluation:** CBC, SMA7 in AM.

Discharge Summary

Patient's Name:
Chart Number:
Date of Admission:
Date of Discharge:
Admitting Diagnosis:
Discharge Diagnosis:
Name of Attending or Ward Service:
Surgical Procedures:
History and Physical Examination and Laboratory Data: Describe the course of the disease up to the time the patient came to the hospital, and describe the physical exam and laboratory data on admission.
Hospital Course: Describe the course of the patient's illness while in the hospital, including evaluation, treatment, outcome of treatment, and medications given.
Discharged Condition: Describe improvement or deterioration in condition.
Disposition: Describe the situation to which the patient will be discharged (home, nursing home).
Discharged Medications: List medications and instructions.
Discharged Instructions and Follow-up Care: Date of return for follow-up care at clinic; diet, exercise instructions.
Problem List: List all active and past problems.
Copies: Send copies to attending physician, clinic, consultants and referring physician.

Surgical Progress Note

Surgical progress notes are written in "SOAP" format.

Example Surgical Progress Note

Date/Time:
Post-operative Day Number:
Problem List: Antibiotic day number, and hyperalimentation day number if applicable. List each surgical problem separately (eg, status-post appendectomy, hypokalemia).
Subjective: Describe how the patient feels in the patient's own words, and give observations about the patient. Indicate any new patient complaints, note the adequacy of pain relief, and passing of flatus or bowel movements. Type of food the patient is tolerating (eg, nothing, clear liquids, regular).
Objective:
    Vital Signs: Maximum temperature (T_{max}) over the past 24 hours. Current temperature, vital signs.
    Intake and Output: Volume of oral and intravenous fluids, volume of urine, stools, drains, and nasogastric output.
    Physical Exam:
        General appearance: Alert, ambulating.
        Heart: Regular rate and rhythm, no murmurs.
        Chest: Clear to auscultation.
        Abdomen: Bowel sounds present, soft, nontender.
        Wound Condition: Comment on the wound condition (eg, clean and dry, good granulation, serosanguinous drainage). Condition of dressings, purulent drainage, granulation tissue, erythema; condition of sutures, dehiscence. Amount and color of drainage
        Lab results: White count, hematocrit, and electrolytes, chest x-ray
Assessment and Plan: Evaluate each numbered problem separately. Note the patient's general condition (eg, improving), pertinent developments, and plans (eg, advance diet to regular, chest x-ray). For each numbered problem, discuss any additional orders and plans for discharge or transfer.

Procedure Note

A procedure note should be written in the chart when a procedure is performed.
Procedure notes are brief operative notes.

Procedure Note

Date and time:
Procedure:
Indications:
Patient Consent: Document that the indications, risks and alternatives to
the procedure were explained to the patient. Note that the patient was
given the opportunity to ask questions and that the patient consented to
the procedure in writing.
Lab tests: Relevant labs, such as the INR and CBC
Anesthesia: Local with 2% lidocaine
Description of Procedure: Briefly describe the procedure, including
sterile prep, anesthesia method, patient position, devices used, anatomic
location of procedure, and outcome.
Complications and Estimated Blood Loss (EBL):
Disposition: Describe how the patient tolerated the procedure.
Specimens: Describe any specimens obtained and labs tests which were
ordered.

Discharge Note

The discharge note should be written in the patient's chart prior to discharge.

Discharge Note

Date/time:
Diagnoses:
Treatment: Briefly describe therapy provided during hospitalization,
including antibiotic therapy, surgery, and cardiovascular drugs.
Studies Performed: Electrocardiograms, CT scan.
Discharge medications:
Follow-up Arrangements:

Postoperative Check

A postoperative check should be completed on the evening after surgery. This check is similar to a daily progress note.

Example Postoperative Check

Date/time:
Postoperative Check
Subjective: Note any of the patient's complaints, and note the adequacy of pain relief.
Objective:
  General appearance:
  Vitals: Maximum temperature in the last 24 hours (T_{max}), current temperature, pulse, respiratory rate, blood pressure.
  Urine Output: If urine output is less than 30cc per hour, more fluids should be infused if the patient is hypovolemic.
  Physical Exam: Chest and abdomen should be examined.
  Chest and lungs:
  Wound Examination: The wound should be examined for excessive drainage or bleeding, condition of drains.
  Drainage Volume: Note the volume and characteristics of drainage from Jackson-Pratt drain or other drains.
  Labs: Post-operative hematocrit value and other labs.
Assessment and Plan: Assess the patient's overall condition and status of wound. Comment on abnormal labs, and discuss treatment and discharge plans.

Total Abdominal Hysterectomy and Bilateral Salpingo-oophorectomy Operative Report

Preoperative Diagnosis: 45 year old female, gravida 3 para 3, with menometrorrhagia unresponsive to medical therapy.
Postoperative Diagnosis: Same as above
Operation: Total abdominal hysterectomy and bilateral salpingo-oophorectomy
Surgeon:
Assistant:
Anesthesia: General endotracheal
Findings At Surgery: Enlarged 10 x 12 cm uterus with multiple fibroids. Normal tubes and ovaries bilaterally. Frozen section revealed benign tissue. All specimens sent to pathology.
Description of Operative Procedure: After obtaining informed consent, the patient was taken to the operating room and placed in the supine position, given general anesthesia, and prepped and draped in sterile fashion.

A Pfannenstiel incision was made 2 cm above the symphysis pubis and extended sharply to the rectus fascia. The fascial incision was bilaterally incised with curved Mayo scissors, and the rectus sheath was separated superiorly and inferiorly by sharp and blunt dissection. The peritoneum was grasped between two Kelly clamps, elevated, and incised with a scalpel. The pelvis was examined with the findings noted above. A Balfour retractor was placed into the incision, and the bowel was packed away with moist laparotomy sponges. Two Kocher clamps were placed on the cornua of the uterus and used for retraction.

The round ligaments on both sides were clamped, sutured with #0 Vicryl, and transected. The anterior leaf of the broad ligament was incised along the bladder reflection to the midline from both sides, and the bladder was gently dissected off the lower uterine segment and cervix with a sponge stick.

The retroperitoneal space was opened and the ureters were identified bilaterally. The infundibulopelvic ligaments on both sides were then doubly clamped, transected, and doubly ligated with #O Vicryl. Excellent hemostasis was observed. The uterine arteries were skelatinized bilaterally, clamped with Heaney clamps, transected, and sutured with #O Vicryl. The uterosacral ligaments were clamped bilaterally, transected, and suture ligated in a similar fashion.

The cervix and uterus was amputated, and the vaginal cuff angles were closed with figure-of-eight stitches of #O Vicryl, and then were transfixed to the ipsilateral cardinal and uterosacral ligament. The vaginal cuff was closed with a series of interrupted #O Vicryl, figure-of-eight sutures. Excellent hemostasis was obtained.

The pelvis was copiously irrigated with warm normal saline, and all sponges and instruments were removed. The parietal peritoneum was closed with running #2-O Vicryl. The fascia was closed with running #O Vicryl. The skin was closed with stables. Sponge, lap, needle, and instrument counts were correct times two. The patient was taken to the recovery room, awake and in stable condition.

Estimated Blood Loss (EBL): 150 cc
Specimens: Uterus, tubes, and ovaries
Drains: Foley to gravity
Fluids: Urine output - 100 cc of clear urine
Complications: None
Disposition: The patient was taken to the recovery room in stable condition.

General Gynecology

Management of the Abnormal Pap Smear

Cervical cancer has an incidence of about 15,700 new cases each year (representing 6% of all cancers), and 4,900 women die of the disease each year. Those at increased risk of preinvasive disease include patients with human-papilloma virus (HPV) infection, those infected with HIV, cigarette smokers, those with multiple sexual partners, and those with previous preinvasive or invasive disease.

I. **Screening for cervical cancer**
   A. Regular Pap smears are recommended for all women who are or have been sexually active and who have a cervix.
   B. Testing should begin when the woman first engages in sexual intercourse. Adolescents whose sexual history is thought to be unreliable should be presumed to be sexually active at age 18.
   C. Pap smears should be performed at least every 1 to 3 years. Testing is usually discontinued after age 65 in women who have had regular normal screening tests. Women who have had a hysterectomy, including removal of the cervix for reasons other than cervical cancer or its precursors, do not require Pap testing.

II. **Management of minor Pap smear abnormalities**
   A. **Satisfactory, but limited by few (or absent) endocervical cells**
      1. Endocervical cells are absent in up to 10% of Pap smears before menopause and up to 50% postmenopausally.
      2. **Management.** The Pap smear is usually either repeated annually or recall women with previously abnormal Pap smears.
   B. **Unsatisfactory for evaluation**
      1. Repeat Pap smear midcycle in 6-12 weeks.
      2. If atrophic smear, treat with estrogen cream for 6-8 weeks, then repeat Pap smear.
   C. **Benign cellular changes**
      1. **Infection--candida.** Most cases represent asymptomatic colonization. Treatment should be offered for symptomatic cases. The Pap should be repeated at the usual interval.
      2. **Infection--Trichomonas.** If wet preparation is positive, treat with metronidazole (Flagyl), then continue annual Pap smears.
      3. **Infection--predominance of coccobacilli consistent with shift in vaginal flora.** This finding implies bacterial vaginosis, but it is a non-specific finding. Diagnosis should be confirmed by findings of a homogeneous vaginal discharge, positive amine test, and clue cells on saline suspension.
      4. **Infection-herpes simplex virus.** Pap smear has a poor sensitivity, but good specificity, for HSV. Positive smears usually are caused by asymptomatic infection. The patient should be informed of pregnancy risks and the possibility of transmission. Treatment is not necessary, and the Pap should be repeated as for a benign result.
      5. **Inflammation on Pap smear**
         a. **Mild inflammation** on an otherwise normal smear does not need further evaluation.
         b. **Moderate or severe inflammation** should be evaluated with a saline preparation, KOH preparation, and gonorrhea and Chlamydia tests. If the source of infection is found, treatment should be provided, and a repeat Pap smear should be done every 6 to 12 months. If no etiology is found, the Pap smear should be repeated in 6 months.
         c. **Persistent inflammation** may be infrequently the only manifestation of high-grade squamous intraepithelial lesions

(HGSIL) or invasive cancer; therefore, persistent inflammation is an indication for colposcopy.

6. **Atrophy with inflammation** is common in post-menopausal women or in those with estrogen-deficiency states. Atrophy should be treated with vaginal estrogen for 4-6 weeks, then repeat Pap smear.

III. **Managing cellular abnormalities**

A. **Atypical squamous cells of undetermined significance (ASCUS).** On retesting, 25%-60% of patients will have LSIL or HSIL, and 15% will demonstrate HSIL. In a low-risk patient, it is reasonable to offer the option of repeating the cervical smears every 4 months for the next 2 years--with colposcopy, endocervical curettage (ECC) and directed biopsy if findings show progression or the atypical cells have not resolved. Alternatively, the patient can proceed immediately with colposcopy, ECC, and directed biopsy. In a high-risk patient (particularly when follow-up may be a problem), it is advisable to proceed with colposcopy, ECC, and directed biopsy.

B. **Low-grade squamous intraepithelial lesion (LSIL).** The smear will revert to normal within 2 years in 30%-60% of patients. Another 25% have, or will progress to, moderate or severe dysplasia (HSIL). With a low-risk patient, cervical smears should be repeated every 4 months for 2 years; colposcopy, ECC, and directed biopsy are indicated for progression or nonresolution. In the high-risk patient, prompt colposcopy, ECC, and directed biopsy are recommended.

The Bethesda system

Adequacy of the specimen
  Satisfactory for evaluation
  Satisfactory for evaluation but limited by... Specify reason
  Unsatisfactory for evaluation: Specify reason
General categorization (optional)
  Within normal limits
  Benign cellular changes: See descriptive diagnoses
  Epithelial cell abnormality: See descriptive diagnoses
Descriptive diagnoses
  Benign cellular changes
  Infection
  Trichomonas vaginalis
  Fungal organisms morphologically consistent with Candida spp
  Predominance of coccobacilli consistent with shift in vaginal flora
  Bacteria morphologically consistent with Actinomyces spp
  Cellular changes associated with herpes simplex virus
  Other
  Reactive changes
  Inflammation (includes typical repair)
  Atrophy with inflammation (atrophic vaginitis)
  Radiation
  Intrauterine contraceptive device
Epithelial cell abnormalities
Squamous cell
  Atypical squamous cells of undetermined significance (ASCUS): Qualify
  Low-grade squamous intraepithelial lesion (LSIL) compassing HPV; mild dysplasia/CIN 1
  High-grade squamous intraepithelial lesions (HSIL) encompassing moderate and severe dysplasia, CIS/CIN 2 and CIN
  Squamous cell carcinoma
Glandular cell
  Endometrial cells, cytologically benign, in a postmenopausal woman
  Atypical glandular cells of undetermined significance (AGUS): Qualify
  Endocervical adenocarcinoma
  Endometrial adenocarcinoma
  Extrauterine adenocarcinoma
  Adenocarcinoma, not otherwise specified
Other malignant neoplasms: Specify

C. **High-grade squamous intraepithelial lesions (HSIL),** moderate-to-severe dysplasia, CIS 1, CIN 2, and CIN 3 Colposcopy, ECC, and directed biopsies are recommended.

D. **Atypical glandular cells of undetermined significance (AGUS).** One-third of those for whom the report "favors reactive" will actually have dysplasia. For this reason, colposcopy, ECC (or cytobrush), and directed biopsies are recommended. If glandular neoplasia is suspected or persistent AGUS does not correlate with ECC findings, cold-knife conization perhaps with dilatation and curettage (D&C) is indicated. D&C with hysteroscopy is the treatment of choice for AGUS endometrial cells.

E. **Squamous cell carcinoma** should be referred to a gynecologist or oncologist experienced in its treatment.

IV. **Management of glandular cell abnormalities**

A. **Endometrial cells on Pap smear.** When a Pap smear is performed during menstruation, endometrial cells may be present. However, endometrial cells on a Pap smear performed during the second half of the menstrual cycle or in a post-menopausal patient may indicate the presence of polyps, hyperplasia, or endometrial adenocarcinoma. An endometrial biopsy should be considered in these women.

B. **Atypical glandular cells of undetermined significance (AGUS).** Colposcopically directed biopsy and endocervical curettage is recommended in all women with AGUS smears, and abnormal endometrial cells should be investigated by endometrial biopsy, fractional curettage, or hysteroscopy.

C. **Adenocarcinoma.** This diagnosis requires endocervical curettage, cone biopsy, and/or endometrial biopsy.

V. **Colposcopically directed biopsy**

A. Liberally apply a solution of 3-5% acetic acid to cervix, and inspect cervix for abnormal areas (white epithelium, punctation, mosaic cells, atypical vessels). Biopsies of any abnormal areas should be obtained under colposcopic visualization. Record location of each biopsy. Monsel solution may be applied to stop bleeding.

B. **Endocervical curettage** is done routinely during colposcopy, except during pregnancy.

VI. **Treatment based on cervical biopsy findings**

A. **Benign cellular changes (infection, reactive inflammation).** Treat the infection, and repeat the smear every 4-6 months; after 2 negatives, repeat yearly.

B. **Squamous intraepithelial lesions**
   1. Women with SIL should be treated on the basis of the histological biopsy diagnosis. Patients with CIN I require no further treatment because the majority of these lesions resolve spontaneously. Patients with CIN II or CIN III require treatment to prevent development of invasive disease.
   2. These lesions are treated with cryotherapy, laser vaporization, or loop electric excision procedure (LEEP).

References: See page 140.

Contraception

One-half of unplanned pregnancies occur among the 10 percent of women who do not use contraception. The remainder of unintended pregnancies result from contraceptive failure.

Advantages and Disadvantages of Various Birth Control Methods		
Method	Advantages	Disadvantages
Diaphragm	Inexpensive; some protection against STDs other than HIV	Not to be used with oil-based lubricants; latex allergy; urinary tract infections
Cervical cap (Prentif Cavit)	Inexpensive; some protection against STDs other than HIV	Damaged by oil-based lubricants; latex allergy; toxic shock syndrome; decreased efficacy with increased frequency of intercourse; difficult to use
Oral combination contraceptive	Decreased menstrual flow and cramping; decreased incidence of pelvic inflammatory disease, ovarian and endometrial cancers, ovarian cyst, ectopic pregnancy, fibrocystic breasts, fibroids, endometriosis and toxic shock syndrome; highly effective	Increased risk of benign hepatic adenomas; mildly increased risk of blood pressure elevation or thromboembolism; no protection against HIV and other STDs; nausea
Depot-medroxy-progesterone acetate (Depo-Provera)	Decreased or no menstrual flow or cramps; compatible with breast-feeding; highly effective	Delayed return of fertility; irregular bleeding; decreased libido; no protection against HIV; nausea
Intrauterine device	Long-term use (up to 10 years)	Increased bleeding, spotting or cramping; risk of ectopic pregnancy with failure; risk of infertility; no protection against HIV and other STDs
Progestin-only agent	Compatible with breast-feeding; no estrogenic side effects	Possible amenorrhea; must be taken at the same time every day; no protection against HIV; nausea
Levonorgestrel implant (Norplant)	Decreased menstrual flow, cramping and ovulatory pain; no adherence requirements; highly effective	Costly; surgical procedure required for insertion; no protection against HIV
Tubal ligation	Low failure rate; no adherence requirements	Surgery; no protection against HIV and other STDs
Vasectomy	Low failure rate; no adherence requirements; outpatient procedure	Surgical procedure; postoperative infection; no protection against HIV

Method	Advantages	Disadvantages
Condoms (male and female)	Inexpensive; some protection against HIV infection and other STDs	Poor acceptance by some users; latex allergy; not to be used with oil-based lubricants

I. **Oral contraceptives**
   A. Two types of oral contraceptives are available in the USA: combination oral contraceptives that contain both an estrogen and a progestin, and progestin-only contraceptives, or "mini-pills." All oral contraceptives marketed in the USA are similarly effective in preventing pregnancy.

Oral Contraceptives		
Drug	**Estrogen (ug)**	**Progestin (mg)**
Monophasic Combination		
Ovral 21, 28	ethinyl estradiol (50)	norgestrel (0.5)
Ogestrel-28	ethinyl estradiol (50)	norgestrel (0.5)
Ovcon 50 28	ethinyl estradiol (50)	norethindrone (1)
Zovia 1/50E 21	ethinyl estradiol (50)	ethynodiol diacetate (1)
Genora 1/50 28	mestranol (50)	norethindrone (1)
Necon 1/50 21, 28	mestranol (50)	norethindrone (1)
Nelova 1/50 21, 28	mestranol (50)	norethindrone (1)
Norinyl 1/50 21, 28	mestranol (50)	norethindrone (1)
Ortho-Novum 1/5028	mestranol (50)	norethindrone (1)
Ovcon 35 21, 28	ethinyl estradiol (35)	norethindrone (0.4)
Brevicon 21, 28	ethinyl estradiol (35)	norethindrone (0.5)
Modicon 28	ethinyl estradiol (35)	norethindrone (0.5)
Necon 0.5/35E 21, 28	ethinyl estradiol (35)	norethindrone (0.5)
Nelova 10/11 21	ethinyl estradiol (35)	norethindrone (0.5, 1)
Genora 1/35 21, 28	ethinyl estradiol (35)	norethindrone (1)
Necon 1/35 21	ethinyl estradiol (35)	norethindrone (1)
Nelova 1/35 28	ethinyl estradiol (35)	norethindrone (1)
Norinyl 1/35 21, 28	ethinyl estradiol (35)	norethindrone (1)
Ortho-Novum 1/35 21, 28	ethinyl estradiol (35)	norethindrone (1)

Ortho-Cyclen* 21, 28	ethinyl estradiol (35)	norgestimate (0.25)
Demulen 1/35 21	ethinyl estradiol (35)	ethynodiol diacetate (1)
Zovia 1/35 E	ethinyl estradiol (35)	ethynodiol diacetate (1)
LoEstrin 1.5/30 21, 28	ethinyl estradiol (30)	norethindrone acetate (1.5)
Levlen 21, 28	ethinyl estradiol (30)	levonorgestrel (0.15)
Levora 21, 28	ethinyl estradiol (30)	levonorgestrel (0.15)
Nordette 21, 28	ethinyl estradiol (30)	levonorgestrel (0.15)
Lo/Ovral	ethinyl estradiol (30)	norgestrel (0.3)
Low-Ogestrel	ethinyl estradiol (30)	norgestrel (0.3)
Desogen* 28	ethinyl estradiol (30)	desogestrel (0.15)
Ortho-Cept* 21	ethinyl estradiol (30)	desogestrel (0.15)
Alesse** 21, 28	ethinyl estradiol (20)	levonorgestrel (0.1)
Levlite** 21, 28	ethinyl estradiol (20)	levonorgestrel (0.1)
LoEstrin** 1/20 21, 28	ethinyl estradiol (20)	norethindrone acetate (1)
Multiphasic Combination		
Tri-Levlen 21, 28	ethinyl estradiol (30, 40, 30)	levonorgestrel (0.05, 0.075, 0.125)
Triphasil 21	ethinyl estradiol (30, 40, 30)	levonorgestrel (0.05, 0.075, 0.125)
Trivora-28	ethinyl estradiol (30, 40, 30)	levonorgestrel (0.05, 0.075, 0.125)
Estrostep 28	ethinyl estradiol (20, 30, 35)	norethindrone acetate (1)
Ortho Tri-Cyclen* 30	ethinyl estradiol (35)	norgestimate (0.18, 0.215, 0.25)
Tri-Norinyl 21, 28	ethinyl estradiol (35)	norethindrone (0.5, 1, 0.5)
Ortho-Novum 7/7/7 21	ethinyl estradiol (35)	norethindrone (0.5, 0.75, 1)
Jenest-28	ethinyl estradiol (35)	norethindrone (0.5, 1)
Necon 10/11 21, 28	ethinyl estradiol (35)	norethindrone (0.5, 1)
Ortho-Novum 10/11 28	ethinyl estradiol (35)	norethindrone (0.5, 1)

Mircette* 28	ethinyl estradiol (20, 0, 10)	desogestrel (0.15)
Progestin Only		
Ovrette		norgestrel (0.075)
Micronor		norethindrone (0.35)
Nor-QD		norethindrone (0.35)

*Third generation agent
**Very low-dose estrogen agent

- B. **Combination oral contraceptives.** Monophasic oral contraceptives contain fixed doses of estrogen and progestin in each active pill. Multiphasic oral contraceptives vary the dose of one or both hormones during the cycle. The rationale for multiphasic oral contraceptives is that they more closely simulate the hormonal changes of a normal menstrual cycle. Multi-phasic pills have a lower total hormone dose per cycle, but there is no convincing evidence that they cause fewer adverse effects or offer any other advantage over monophasic pills, which are simpler to take.
- C. **Adverse effects.** Estrogens can cause nausea, breast tenderness and breast enlargement. Progestins can cause unfavorable changes in LDL and HDL cholesterol. Other adverse effects associated with oral contraceptives, such as weight gain or depression, are more difficult to attribute to one component or the other. Women smokers more than 35 years old who use combination oral contraceptives have an increased risk of cardiovascular disease.
- D. **Acne.** Use of a combined oral contraceptive containing norgestimate (Ortho Tri-Cyclen) will often significantly improve acne. Combination oral contraceptives containing levonorgestrel or norethindrone acetate also improved acne.
- E. **Third-generation progestins** (desogestrel, norgestimate, gestodene) used in combination oral contraceptives have been claimed to be less androgenic. They have been associated with a small increase in the risk of venous thromboembolism.
- F. **Very low-dose estrogen.** Combined oral contraceptive products containing 20 μg of ethinyl estradiol may cause less bloating and breast tenderness than those containing higher doses of estrogen. The potential disadvantage of low estrogen doses is more breakthrough bleeding.
- G. **Drug interactions.** Macrolide antibiotics, tetracyclines, rifampin, metronidazole (Flagyl), penicillins, trimethoprim-sulfamethoxazole (Bactrim), several anti-HIV agents and many anti-epileptic drugs, can induce the metabolism and decrease the effectiveness of oral contraceptives.
- H. A careful personal and family medical history (with particular attention to cardiovascular risk factors) and an accurate blood pressure measurement are recommended before the initiation of oral contraceptive pills. A physical examination and a Papanicolaou smear (with screening genital cultures as indicated) are usually performed at the time oral contraceptive pills are initially prescribed. An initial prescription of OCPs can be written before a physical examination and a Pap test are performed in healthy young women.

Noncontraceptive Benefits of Oral Contraceptive Pills

Dysmenorrhea Mittelschmerz
Metrorrhagia
Premenstrual syndrome
Hirsutism
Ovarian and endometrial cancer

Functional ovarian cysts
Benign breast cysts
Ectopic pregnancy
Acne
Endometriosis

Factors to Consider in Starting or Switching Oral Contraceptive Pills

Objective	Action	Products that achieve the objective
To minimize high risk of thrombosis	Select a product with a lower dosage of estrogen.	Alesse, Loestrin 1/20, Levlite, Mircette
To minimize nausea, breast tenderness or vascular headaches	Select a product with a lower dosage of estrogen.	Alesse, Levlite, Loestrin 1/20, Mircette
To minimize spotting or breakthrough bleeding	Select a product with a higher dosage of estrogen or a progestin with greater potency.	Demulen, Desogen, Levlen, Lo/Ovral, Nordette, Ortho-Cept, Ortho-Cyclen, Ortho Tri-Cyclen
To minimize androgenic effects	Select a product containing a third-generation progestin, low-dose norethindrone or ethynodiol diacetate.	Brevicon, Demulen 1/35, Desogen,* Modicon, Ortho-Cept,* Ortho-Cyclen,* Ortho Tri-Cyclen,* Ovcon 35
To avoid dyslipidemia	Select a product containing a third-generation progestin, low-dose norethindrone or ethynodiol diacetate.	Brevicon, Demulen 1/35, Desogen,* Modicon, Ortho-Cept,* Ortho-Cyclen,* Ortho Tri-Cyclen,* Ovcon 35

*--These products contain a third-generation progestin.

Instructions on the Use of Oral Contraceptive Pills

Initiation of use (choose one):
The patient begins taking the pills on the first day of menstrual bleeding.
The patient begins taking the pills on the first Sunday after menstrual bleeding begins.
The patient begins taking the pills immediately if she is definitely not pregnant and has not had unprotected sex since her last menstrual period.

Missed pill
If it has been less than 24 hours since the last pill was taken, the patient takes a pill right away and then returns to normal pill-taking routine.
If it has been 24 hours since the last pill was taken, the patient takes both the missed pill and the next scheduled pill at the same time.
If it has been more than 24 hours since the last pill was taken (ie, two or more missed pills), the patient takes the last pill that was missed, throws out the other missed pills and takes the next pill on time. Additional contraception is used for the remainder of the cycle.

Additional contraceptive method
The patient uses an additional contraceptive method for the first 7 days after initially starting oral contraceptive pills.
The patient uses an additional contraceptive method for 7 days if she is more than 12 hours late in taking an oral contraceptive pill.
The patient uses an additional contraceptive method while she is taking an interacting drug and for 7 days thereafter.

Contraindications to Use of Hormonal Contraceptive Methods

Method	Contraindications
Oral combination contraceptive	Active liver disease, hepatic adenoma, thrombophlebitis, history of or active thromboembolic disorder, cardiovascular or cerebrovascular disease, known or suspected breast cancer, undiagnosed abnormal vaginal bleeding, jaundice with past pregnancy or hormone use, pregnancy, breast-feeding, smoking in women over age 35
Progestin-only pill	Undiagnosed abnormal vaginal bleeding, known or suspected breast cancer, cholestatic jaundice of pregnancy or jaundice with previous pill use, hepatic adenoma, known or suspected pregnancy
Depot-medroxyprogester-one acetate (Depo-Provera) injection	Acute liver disease or tumor, thrombophlebitis, known or suspected breast cancer, undiagnosed abnormal vaginal bleeding
Levonorgestrel implant (Norplant)	Acute liver disease or tumor, active thrombophlebitis, known or suspected breast cancer, history of idiopathic intracranial hypertension, undiagnosed abnormal vaginal bleeding, pregnancy, hypersensitivity to any component of the implant system

Side Effects of Hormones Used in Contraceptive Agents

Type of effect	Symptoms
Estrogenic	Nausea, breast tenderness, fluid retention
Progestational	Acne, increased appetite, weight gain, depression, fatigue
Androgenic	Weight gain. hirsutism, acne, oily skin, breakthrough bleeding

I. **Administration issues**
   1. **Amenorrhea** may occur with long-term use. Administration of an agent with higher estrogen or lower progestin activity may resolve this problem. A missed menstrual period indicates a need for a pregnancy test.
   2. **Breakthrough bleeding** often occurs during the first three months of use. If breakthrough bleeding is a problem, a higher-dose progestin or estrogen agent may be tried. Agents that contain norgestrel are associated with low rates of breakthrough bleeding.

J. **Progestin-only agents**
   1. Progestin-only agents are slightly less effective than combination oral contraceptives. They have failure rates of 0.5 percent compared with the 0.1 percent rate with combination oral contraceptives.
   2. Progestin-only oral contraceptives (Micronor, Nor-QD, Ovrette) provide

a useful alternative in women who cannot take estrogen and those over age 40. Progestin-only contraception is recommended for nursing mothers. Milk production is unaffected by use of progestin-only agents.

3. If the usual time of ingestion is delayed for more than three hours, an alternative form of birth control should be used for the following 48 hours. Because progestin-only agents are taken continuously, without hormone-free periods, menses may be irregular, infrequent or absent.

II. Medroxyprogesterone acetate injections

A. Depot medroxyprogesterone acetate (Depo-Provera) is an injectable progestin. A 150-mg dose provides 12 weeks of contraception. However, an effective level of contraception is maintained for 14 weeks after an injection. After discontinuation of the injections, resumption of ovulation may require up to nine months.

B. The medication is given IM every 12 weeks. An injection should be administered within five days after the onset of menses or after proof of a negative pregnancy test. Medroxyprogesterone may be administered immediately after childbirth.

C. Medroxyprogesterone injections are a good choice for patients, such as adolescents, who have difficulty remembering to take their oral contraceptive or who have a tendency to use other methods inconsistently. Medroxyprogesterone may also be a useful choice for women who have contraindications to estrogen. This method should not be used for women who desire a rapid return to fertility after discontinuing contraception.

D. **Contraindications and side effects**
  1. Breakthrough bleeding is common during the first few months of use. Most women experience regular bleeding or amenorrhea within six months after the first injection. If breakthrough bleeding persists beyond this period, nonsteroidal anti-inflammatory agents, combination oral contraceptives or a 10- to 21-day course of oral estrogen may eliminate the problem. About 50% of women who have received the injections for one year experience amenorrhea.
  2. Side effects include weight gain, headache and dizziness.

III. Diaphragm

A. Diaphragms function as a physical barrier and as a reservoir for spermicide. They are particularly acceptable for patients who have only intermittent intercourse. Diaphragms are available in 5-mm incremental sizes from 55 to 80 mm. They must remain in place for eight hours after intercourse and may be damaged by oil-based lubricants.

B. **Method for fitting a diaphragm**
  1. Selecting a diaphragm may begin by inserting a 70-mm diaphragm (the average size) and then determining whether this size is correct or is too large or too small.
  2. Another method is to estimate the appropriate size by placing a gloved hand in the vagina and using the index and middle fingers to measure the distance from the introitus to the cervix.

IV. Levonorgestrel contraceptive implant (Norplant) is effective for 5 years and consists of six flexible Silastic capsules. Adequate serum levels are obtained within 24 hours after implantation.

V. Emergency contraception

A. Emergency contraception may be considered for a patient who reports a contraceptive failure, such as condom breakage, or other circumstances of unprotected sexual intercourse, such as a sexual assault. If menstruation does not occur within 21 days, a pregnancy test should be performed.

B. Emergency contraception is effective for up to 72 hours after intercourse.

Emergency Contraception

1. Consider pretreatment one hour before each oral contraceptive pill dose, using one of the following orally administered antiemetic agents:
   Prochlorperazine (Compazine), 5 to 10 mg
   Promethazine (Phenergan), 12.5 to 25 mg
   Trimethobenzamide (Tigan), 250 mg
2. Administer the first dose of oral contraceptive pill within 72 hours of unprotected coitus, and administer the second dose 12 hours after the first dose. Brand name options for emergency contraception include the following:
   Preven Kit--two pills per dose (0.5 mg of levonorgestrel and 100 µg of ethinyl estradiol per dose) Ovral--two pills per dose (0.5 mg of levonorgestrel and 100 µg of ethinyl estradiol per dose)
   Nordette--four pills per dose (0.6 mg of levonorgestrel and 120 µg of ethinyl estradiol per dose)
   Triphasil--four pills per dose (0.5 mg of levonorgestrel and 120 µg of ethinyl estradiol per dose)
   Plan B--one pill per dose (0.75 mg of levonorgestrel per dose)

   C. The major side effect of emergency contraception with oral contraceptives is nausea, which occurs in 50% of women; vomiting occurs in 20%. If the patient vomits within two hours after ingesting a dose, the dose should be repeated. An antiemetic, such as phenothiazine (Compazine), 5-10 mg PO, or trimethobenzamide (Tigan), 100-250 mg, may be taken one hour before administration of the contraceptive.

  VI. **Intrauterine devices**
   A. IUDs represent the most commonly used method of reversible contraception worldwide. The Progestasert IUD releases progesterone and must be replaced every 12 months. The Copper-T IUD is a copper-containing device which may be used for 10 years.
   B. IUDs act by causing a localized foreign-body inflammatory reaction that inhibits implantation of the ovum. An IUD may be a good choice for parous women who are in a monogamous relationship and do not have dysmenorrhea.
   C. **Contraindications** include women who are at high risk for STDs and those who have a history of pelvic inflammatory disease, and women at high risk for endocarditis. Oral administration of doxycycline, 200 mg, or azithromycin (Zithromax), 500 mg, one hour before insertion reduces the incidence of insertion-related infections.

References: See page 140.

Pregnancy Termination

Ninety percent of abortions are performed in the first trimester of pregnancy. About 1.5 million legal abortions are performed each year in the United States. Before 16 weeks of gestation, legal abortion may be performed in an office setting. Major anomalies and mid-trimester premature rupture of membranes are recognized fetal indications for termination.

I. **Menstrual extraction**
   A. Many women seek abortion services within 1-2 weeks of the missed period. Abortion of these early pregnancies with a small-bore vacuum cannula is called menstrual extraction or minisuction. The only instruments required are a speculum, a tenaculum, a Karman cannula, and a modified 50 mL syringe.
   B. The extracted tissue is rinsed and examined in a clear dish of water or

saline over a light source to detect chorionic villi and the gestational sac. This examination is performed to rule out ectopic pregnancy and to decrease the risk of incomplete abortion.

II. First-trimester vacuum curettage

A. Beyond 7 menstrual weeks of gestation, larger cannulas and vacuum sources are required to evacuate a pregnancy. Vacuum curettage is the most common method of abortion. Procedures performed before 13 menstrual weeks are called suction or vacuum curettage, whereas similar procedures carried out after 13 weeks are termed dilation and evacuation.

B. Technique

1. Uterine size and position should be assessed during a pelvic examination before the procedure. Ultrasonography is advised if there is a discrepancy of more than 2 weeks between the uterine size and menstrual dating.

2. Tests for gonorrhea and chlamydia should be obtained, and the cervix and vagina should be prepared with a germicide. Paracervical block is established with 20 mL of 1% lidocaine injected deep into the cervix at the 3, 5, 7, and 9 o'clock positions. The cervix should be grasped with a single-toothed tenaculum placed vertically with one branch inside the canal. Uterine depth is measured with a sound. Dilation then should be performed with a tapered dilator.

3. A vacuum cannula with a diameter in millimeters that is one less than the estimated gestational age should be used to evacuate the cavity. After the tissue is removed, there should be a quick check with a sharp curette, followed by a brief reintroduction of the vacuum cannula. The aspirated tissue should be examined as described previously.

4. Antibiotics are used prophylactically. Doxycycline is the best agent because of a broad spectrum of antimicrobial effect. D-negative patients should receive D (Rho[D]) immune globulin.

C. Complications

1. The most common postabortal complications are pain, bleeding, and low-grade fever. Most cases are caused by retained gestational tissue or a clot in the uterine cavity. These symptoms are best managed by a repeat uterine evacuation, performed under local anesthesia

2. **Cervical shock.** Vasovagal syncope produced by stimulation of the cervical canal can be seen after paracervical block. Brief tonic-clonic activity rarely may be observed and is often confused with seizure. The routine use of atropine with paracervical anesthesia or the use of conscious sedation prevents cervical shock.

3. **Perforation**

   a. The risk of perforation is less than 1 in every 1,000 first-trimester abortions. It increases with gestational age and is greater for parous women than for nulliparous women. Perforation is best evaluated by laparoscopy to determine the extent of the injury.

   b. Perforations at the junction of the cervix and lower uterine segment can lacerate the ascending branch of the uterine artery within the broad ligament, giving rise to severe pain, a broad ligament hematoma, and intraabdominal bleeding. Management requires laparotomy, ligation of the severed vessels, and repair of the uterine injury.

4. **Hemorrhage**

   a. Excessive bleeding may indicate uterine atony, a low-lying implantation, a pregnancy of more advanced gestational age than the first trimester, or perforation. Management requires rapid reassessment of gestational age by examination of the fetal parts already extracted and gentle exploration of the uterine cavity with a curette and forceps. Intravenous oxytocin should be administered, and the abortion should be completed. The uterus then should be massaged to ensure contraction.

   b. When these measures fail, the patient should be hospitalized and should receive intravenous fluids and have her blood crossmatched. Persistent postabortal bleeding strongly suggests retained tissue or clot (hematometra) or trauma, and laparoscopy and repeat vacuum curettage is indicated.

5. **Hematometra.** Lower abdominal pain of increasing intensity in the first 30 minutes suggests hematometra. If there is no fever or bleeding is brisk, and on examination the uterus is large, globular, and tense, hematometra is likely. The treatment is immediate reevacuation.

6. **Ectopic pregnancy incomplete abortion, and failed abortion**

   a. Early detection of ectopic pregnancy, incomplete abortion, or failed abortion is possible with examination of the specimen immediately after the abortion. The patient may have an ectopic pregnancy if no chorionic villi are found. To detect an incomplete abortion that might result in continued pregnancy, the actual gestational sac must be identified. Determination of the b-hCG level and frozen section of the aspirated tissue and vaginal ultrasonography may be useful. If the b-hCG level is greater than 1,500-2,000 mIU, chorionic villi are not identified on frozen section, or retained tissue is identified by ultrasonography, immediate laparoscopy should be considered. Other patients may be followed closely with serial b-hCG assays until the problem is resolved. With later (>13 weeks) gestations, all of the fetal parts must be identified by the surgeon to prevent incomplete abortion.

   b. Heavy bleeding or fever after abortion suggests retained tissue. If the postabortal uterus is larger than 12-week size, preoperative ultrasonography should be performed to determine the amount of remaining tissue. When fever is present, high-dose intravenous antibiotic therapy with two or three agents should be initiated, and curettage should be performed shortly thereafter.

III. **Medical abortion in the first trimester**

A. **Mifepristone (RU 486)** blocks the progesterone receptor. It can effectively induce an abortion in an early gestation after a single oral dose, with an effectiveness of 95%. An oral dose of mifepristone is given on day 1. On day 3, the patient returns for prostaglandin (sulprostone or gemeprost) and D immune globulin if she is D negative. Patients remain in the clinic for 4 hours, during which time expulsion of the pregnancy usually occurs. The patient then returns 8-15 days later for measurement of b-hCG or ultrasonography.

B. **Methotrexate with misoprostol** is also an effective medical regimen for early abortion. Methotrexate is given as a single intramuscular dose followed 5-7 days later with vaginal misoprostol. Efficacy is slightly less than that observed with the mifepristone and misoprostol and bleeding may last longer.

IV. **Second-trimester abortion.** Most abortions are performed before 13 menstrual weeks. Later abortions are generally performed because of fetal defects, maternal illness, or maternal age.

A. **Dilation and evacuation**

1. Transcervical dilation and evacuation of the uterus (D&E) is the method most commonly used for mid-trimester abortions before 21 menstrual weeks. In the one-stage technique, forcible dilation is performed slowly and carefully to sufficient diameter to allow insertion of large, strong ovum forceps for evacuation. The better approach is a two-stage procedure in which multiple Laminaria are used to achieve gradual dilatation over several hours before extraction. Uterine evacuation is accomplished with long, heavy forceps, using the vacuum cannula to rupture the fetal membranes, drain amniotic fluid, and ensure complete evacuation.

2. Preoperative ultrasonography is necessary for all cases 14 weeks and beyond. Intraoperative real-time ultrasonography helps to locate fetal parts within the uterus.

3. Dilation and evacuation becomes progressively more difficult as gestational age advances, and instillation techniques are often used after 21 weeks. Dilation and evacuation can be offered in the late mid-

trimester, but two sets of Laminaria tents for a total of 36-48 hours is recommended. After multistage Laminaria treatment, urea is injected into the amniotic sac. Extraction is then accomplished after labor begins and after fetal maceration has occurred.

References: See page 140.

Ectopic Pregnancy

Ectopic pregnancy causes 15% of all maternal deaths. Once a patient has had an ectopic pregnancy, there is a 7- to 13-fold increase in the risk of recurrence. Factors that have been shown to increase the risk of tubal pregnancy include 1) previous pelvic inflammatory disease, 2) previous tubal surgery, 3) current use of an intrauterine device, and 4) previous ectopic gestation.

I. Evaluation
   A. Any pregnancy in which the embryo implants outside the uterine cavity is defined as an ectopic pregnancy (EP). Hemorrhagic shock secondary to EP accounts for 6-7% of all maternal deaths.

Risk Factors for Ectopic Pregnancy
Lesser Risk Previous pelvic or abdominal surgery Cigarette smoking Vaginal douching Age of 1st intercourse <18 years
Greater Risk Previous genital infections (eg, PID) Infertility (In vitro fertilization) Multiple sexual partners
Greatest Risk Previous ectopic pregnancy Previous tubal surgery or sterilization Diethylstilbestrol exposure in utero Documented tubal pathology (scarring) Use of intrauterine contraceptive device

II. Clinical presentation
   A. The first symptoms of ectopic pregnancy (EP) are those associated with early pregnancy, including nausea with or without vomiting, breast tenderness, and amenorrhea. Nonspecific abdominal pain or pelvic pain is reported in 80% of patients with EP. Patients may also report having "normal" periods, light periods, or spotting.
   B. As an EP progresses, the greatest danger to the patient is fallopian tube rupture. The symptoms of rupture produce the "classical" presentation of sudden, severe unilateral abdominal pain, vaginal bleeding, and a history of amenorrhea.
   C. Classical symptoms are uncommon. Loss of blood into the peritoneal cavity usually will produce symptoms of peritoneal irritation. The uterus in a patient with suspected EP should be softened and normal size, or slightly enlarged but smaller than expected by gestational dates. This finding is reported in up to 70% of cases.

Presenting Signs and Symptoms of Ectopic Pregnancy	
Symptom	**Percentage of Women with Symptom**
Abdominal pain	80-100%
Amenorrhea	75-95%
Vaginal bleeding	50-80%
Dizziness, fainting	20-35%
Urge to defecate	5-15%
Pregnancy symptoms	10-25%
Passage of tissue	5-10%
Sign	**Percentage of Women with Sign**
Adnexal tenderness	75-90%
Abdominal tenderness	80-95%
Adnexal mass	50%
Uterine enlargement	20-30%
Orthostatic changes	10-15%
Fever	5-10%

III. Diagnostic strategy

A. Rh status must be verified in every patient with vaginal bleeding to avoid the failure to treat Rh-negative mothers with Rhogam.

B. Beta-human chorionic gonadotropin
  1. Beta-hCG is a hormone produced by both ectopic and normally implanted trophoblastic cells. Monoclonal antibody assays can detect the presence of beta-hCG as soon as 2-3 days postimplantation. In a normal pregnancy, the level of this protein doubles about every two days up to a value of 10,000 mIU/mL. A urine pregnancy test is ordered to verify the presence of beta-hCG in the urine and, if positive, a serum quantitative level may then be obtained in order to verify if the level is above the discriminatory level for ultrasound.
  2. An intrauterine pregnancy should be seen by transabdominal ultrasound with beta-hCG levels of 6500 mIU/mL, or at 1500 to 2000 mIU/mL using transvaginal ultrasound. Consequently, absence of a gestational sac in a patient whose beta-hCG indicates that a pregnancy should be detectable by these ultrasonographic modalities increases the likelihood for EP. The beta-hCG can be followed in stable patients in whom the level is too low to expect ultrasound visualization of a normal intrauterine pregnancy. The level should be rechecked in 48 hours.

C. Progesterone is produced by the corpus luteum in response to the presence of a pregnancy. Progesterone levels change little in the first 8-10 weeks of gestation. Progesterone levels normally fall after 10 weeks gestation. When a pregnancy fails during the first 8-10 weeks, progesterone levels fall. A single progesterone level higher than 25 ng/mL is consistent with a viable intrauterine pregnancy, and this level excludes EP with a 97.5% sensitivity. Moreover, 25% of viable intrauterine pregnancies have levels below 25 ng/mL. A level below 5 ng/mL is 100% diagnostic of a non-viable pregnancy. However, a low level does not correlate with the location of the pregnancy.

D. Ultrasound
  1. Transvaginal ultrasound has become the single most valuable modality for the work-up of patients suspected of having an EP. The beta-hCG

level at which signs of pregnancy can first be seen ultrasonographically is called the discriminatory threshold.
   2. The discriminatory beta-hCG threshold is between 1000 mIU/mL and 2000 mIU/mL. Transvaginal ultrasound has the capability, assuming sufficiently high and "discriminatory" beta-HCG levels are detected, to identify a pregnancy location as soon as one week after missing a menstrual period.

   E. **Other diagnostic tests**
   1. **Uterine curettage** is performed only when serum hormones indicate a non-viable pregnancy (progesterone <5 ng/mL or falling/plateauing beta-hCG). Typically, chorionic villi are identified (by floating tissue obtained in saline) when a failed intrauterine pregnancy is present. When villi are not seen, diagnosis of completed miscarriage can still be made if the beta-hCG level falls 15% or more 8-12 hours after the procedure. When no villi are seen and beta-hCG levels do not fall, EP is highly suspected. Ectopic pregnancy is diagnosed in this situation if the beta-hCG plateaus or continues to rise after the procedure.
   2. **Laparoscopy** can be both diagnostic and therapeutic for EP. Use of laparoscopy is indicated in patients with peritoneal signs and equivocal results from testing with ultrasound or uterine curettage. It can also used alone for treatment when the diagnosis has been made by other means, although many patients are now managed medically.

IV. **Treatment**
   A. Ectopic pregnancy can be treated medically or surgically.

Criteria for Receiving Methotrexate

Absolute indications
Hemodynamically stable without active bleeding or signs of hemoperitoneum
Nonlaparoscopic diagnosis
Patient desires future fertility
General anesthesia poses a significant risk
Patient is able to return for follow-up care
Patient has no contraindications to methotrexate

Relative indications
Unruptured mass <3.5 cm at its greatest dimension
No fetal cardiac motion detected
Patients whose bet-hCG level does not exceed 6,000-15,000 mIU/mL

Contraindications to Medical Therapy

Absolute contraindications
Breast feeding
Overt or laboratory evidence of immunodeficiency
Alcoholism, alcoholic liver disease, or other chronic liver disease
Preexisting blood dyscrasias, such as bone marrow hypoplasia, leukopenia, thrombocytopenia, or significant anemia
Known sensitivity to methotrexate
Active pulmonary disease
Peptic ulcer disease
Hepatic, renal, or hematologic dysfunction
Relative contraindications
Gestational sac >3.5 cm
Embryonic cardiac motion

   B. **Methotrexate**
   1. Before methotrexate is injected, blood is drawn to determine baseline laboratory values for renal, liver, bone marrow function, beta-hCG level, and progesterone Blood type, Rh factor, and the presence of antibodies should be determined. Patients who are Rh negative should receive Rh

immune globulin.

2. **The methotrexate dose** is calculated according to estimated body surface area (50 mg/m^2) and is given in one dose. Treatment with a standard 75 mg dose and multiple serial doses with a folinic acid rescue on alternate days (four doses of methotrexate [1.0 mg/kg] on days 0, 2, 4, and 6 and four doses of leucovorin [0.1 mg/kg] on days 1, 3, 5, and 7) also have been successful.

3. **Follow-up care** continues until beta-hCG levels are nondetectable. Time to resolution is variable and can be protracted, taking a month or longer. With the single-dose regimen, levels of beta-hCG usually increase during the first several days following methotrexate injection and peak 4 days after injection. If a treatment response is observed, hCG levels should decline by 7 days after injection. If the beta-hCG level does not decline by at least 15% from day 4 to day 7, the patient may require either surgery, or a second dose of methotrexate. If there is an adequate treatment response, hCG determinations are reduced to once a week. An additional dose of methotrexate may be given if beta-hCG levels plateau or increase in 7 days.

4. **Surgical intervention** may be required for patients who do not respond to medical therapy. Ultrasound examination may be repeated to evaluate increased pelvic pain, bleeding, or inadequate declines of beta-hCG levels.

Side Effects Associated with Methotrexate Treatment

Nausea	Vaginal bleeding or spotting
Vomiting	Severe neutropenia (rare)
Stomatitis	Reversible alopecia (rare)
Diarrhea	Pneumonitis
Gastric distress	Treatment effects
Dizziness	Increase in abdominal pain (occurs in
Increase in beta-hCG levels during first	up to two-thirds of patients)
1-3 days of treatment	

Signs of treatment failure and tubal rupture

Significantly worsening abdominal pain, regardless of change in beta-hCG levels
Hemodynamic instability
Levels of beta-hCG that do not decline by at least 15% between day 4 and day 7 postinjection
Increasing or plateauing beta-hCG levels after the first week of treatment

5. During treatment, patients should be counseled to discontinue folinic acid supplements, including prenatal vitamins, and avoid the use of nonsteroidal antiinflammatory drugs.

6. An initial increase in beta-hCG levels often occurs by the third day and is not a cause for alarm. Most patients experience at least one episode of increased abdominal pain sometime during treatment. Abdominal pain may also suggest tubal rupture.

7. Medical treatment has failed when beta-hCG levels either increase or plateau by day 7, indicating a continuing ectopic pregnancy, or when the tube ruptures.

C. **Operative management** can be accomplished by either laparoscopy or laparotomy. Linear salpingostomy or segmental resection is the procedure of choice if the fallopian tube is to be retained. Salpingectomy is the procedure of choice if the tube requires removal.

References: See page 140.

Acute Pelvic Pain

I. **Clinical evaluation**
   A. Assessment of acute pelvic pain should determine the patient's age, obstetrical history, menstrual history, characteristics of pain onset, duration, and palliative or aggravating factors.
   B. **Associated symptoms** may include urinary or gastrointestinal symptoms, fever, abnormal bleeding, or vaginal discharge.
   C. **Past medical history.** Contraceptive history, surgical history, gynecologic history, history of pelvic inflammatory disease, ectopic pregnancy, sexually transmitted diseases should be determined. Current sexual activity and practices should be assessed.
   D. **Method of contraception**
      1. Sexual abstinence in the months preceding the onset of pain lessons the likelihood of pregnancy-related etiologies.
      2. The risk of acute PID is reduced by 50% in patients taking oral contraceptives or using a barrier method of contraception. Patients taking oral contraceptives are at decreased risk for an ectopic pregnancy or ovarian cysts.
   E. **Risk factors for acute pelvic inflammatory disease.** Age between 15-25 years, sexual partner with symptoms of urethritis, prior history of PID.

II. **Physical examination**
   A. Fever, abdominal or pelvic tenderness, and peritoneal signs should be sought.
   B. Vaginal discharge, cervical erythema and discharge, cervical and uterine motion tenderness, or adnexal masses or tenderness should be noted.

III. **Laboratory tests**
   A. **Pregnancy testing** will identify pregnancy-related causes of pelvic pain. Serum beta-HCG becomes positive 7 days after conception. A negative test virtually excludes ectopic pregnancy.
   B. **Complete blood count.** Leukocytosis suggest an inflammatory process; however, a normal white blood count occurs in 56% of patients with PID and 37% of patients with appendicitis.
   C. **Urinalysis.** The finding of pyuria suggests urinary tract infection. Pyuria can also occur with an inflamed appendix or from contamination of the urine by vaginal discharge.
   D. **Testing for Neisseria gonorrhoeae and Chlamydia trachomatis** are necessary if PID is a possibility.
   E. **Pelvic ultrasonography** is of value in excluding the diagnosis of an ectopic pregnancy by demonstrating an intrauterine gestation. Sonography may reveal acute PID, torsion of the adnexa, or acute appendicitis.
   F. **Diagnostic laparoscopy** is indicated when acute pelvic pain has an unclear diagnosis despite comprehensive evaluation.

III. **Differential diagnosis of acute pelvic pain**
   A. **Pregnancy-related causes.** Ectopic pregnancy, spontaneous, threatened or incomplete abortion, intrauterine pregnancy with corpus luteum bleeding.
   B. **Gynecologic disorders.** PID, endometriosis, ovarian cyst hemorrhage or rupture, adnexal torsion, Mittelschmerz, uterine leiomyoma torsion, primary dysmenorrhea, tumor.
   C. **Nonreproductive tract causes**
      1. **Gastrointestinal.** Appendicitis, inflammatory bowel disease, mesenteric adenitis, irritable bowel syndrome, diverticulitis.
      2. **Urinary tract.** Urinary tract infection, renal calculus.

IV. **Approach to acute pelvic pain with a positive pregnancy test**
   A. In a female patient of reproductive age, presenting with acute pelvic pain, the first distinction is whether the pain is pregnancy-related or non-pregnancy-related on the basis of a serum pregnancy test.
   B. In the patient with acute pelvic pain associated with pregnancy, the next step is localization of the tissue responsible for the hCG production. Transvaginal ultrasound should be performed to identify an intrauterine

gestation. Ectopic pregnancy is characterized by a noncystic adnexal mass and fluid in the cul-de-sac.

C. **If a gestational sac is not demonstrated on ultrasonography, the following possibilities exist:**
   1. **Ectopic pregnancy**
   2. **Very early intrauterine pregnancy** not seen on ultrasound
   3. **Recent abortion**
D. **Management of patients when a gestational sac is not seen with a positive pregnancy test**
   1. **Diagnostic laparoscopy** is the most accurate and rapid method of establishing or excluding the diagnosis of ectopic pregnancy.
   2. **Examination of endometrial tissue.** For pregnant patients desiring termination, and for those patients in whom it can be demonstrated that the pregnancy is nonviable, suction curettage with immediate histologic examination of the curettings is a diagnostic option. The presence of chorionic villi confirms the diagnosis of intrauterine pregnancy, whereas the absence of such villi indicates ectopic pregnancy.

V. **Management of the ectopic gestation**
   A. Two IV catheters of at least 18 gauge should be placed and 1-2 L of normal saline infused.
   B. **Laparoscopy or laparotomy** with linear salpingostomy or salpingectomy should be accomplished in unstable patients. An HCG level should be checked in one week to assure that the level is declining.
   C. **Methotrexate.** Stable patients can be treated with methotrexate in a single intramuscular dose of 50 mg per meter^2. Treatment response should be assessed by serial HCG measurements made until the hormone is undetectable.

VI. **Approach to acute pelvic pain in non-pregnant patients with a negative HCG**
   A. **Acute PID** is the leading diagnostic consideration in patients with acute pelvic pain unrelated to pregnancy. The pain is usually bilateral, but may be unilateral in 10%. Cervical motion tenderness, fever, and cervical discharge are common findings.
   B. **Acute appendicitis** should be considered in all patients presenting with acute pelvic pain and a negative pregnancy test. Appendicitis is characterized by leukocytosis and a history of a few hours of periumbilical pain followed by migration of the pain to the right lower quadrant. Neutrophilia occurs in 75%. A slight fever exceeding 37.3°C, nausea, vomiting, anorexia, and rebound tenderness may be present.
   C. **Torsion of the adnexa** usually causes unilateral pain, but pain can be bilateral in 25%. Intense, progressive pain combined with a tense, tender adnexal mass is characteristic. There is often a history of repetitive, transitory pain. Pelvic sonography often confirms the diagnosis. Laparoscopic diagnosis and surgical intervention are indicated.
   D. **Ruptured or hemorrhagic corpus luteal cyst** usually causes bilateral pain, but it can cause unilateral tenderness in 35%. Ultrasound aids in diagnosis.
   E. **Endometriosis** usually causes chronic or recurrent pain, but it can occasionally cause acute pelvic pain. There usually is a history of dysmenorrhea and deep dyspareunia. Pelvic exam reveals fixed uterine retrodisplacement and tender uterosacral and cul-de-sac nodularity. Laparoscopy confirms the diagnosis.

References: See page 140.

Chronic Pelvic Pain

Chronic pelvic pain (CPP) affects approximately one in seven women in the United States (14 percent). Chronic pelvic pain (>6 months in duration) is less likely to be associated with a readily identifiable cause than is acute pain.

32 Chronic Pelvic Pain

I. Etiology of chronic pelvic pain

A. Physical and sexual abuse.
Numerous studies have demonstrated a higher frequency of physical and/or sexual abuse in women with CPP. Between 30 and 50 percent of women with CPP have a history of abuse (physical or sexual, childhood or adult).

B. Gynecologic problems

1. **Endometriosis** is present in approximately one-third of women undergoing laparoscopy for CPP and is the most frequent finding in these women. Typically, endometriosis pain is a sharp or "crampy" pain. It starts at the onset of menses, becoming more severe and prolonged over several menstrual cycles. It is frequently accompanied by deep dyspareunia. Uterosacral ligament nodularity is highly specific for endometriosis. Examining the woman during her menstruation may make the nodularity easier to palpate. A more common, but less specific, finding is tenderness in the cul-de-sac or uterosacral ligaments that reproduces the pain of deep dyspareunia.

2. **Pelvic adhesions** are found in approximately one-fourth of women undergoing laparoscopy for CPP. Adhesions form after intra-abdominal inflammation; they should be suspected if the woman has a history of surgery or pelvic inflammatory disease (PID). The pain may be a dull or sharp pulling sensation that occurs at any time during the month. Physical examination is usually nondiagnostic.

3. **Dysmenorrhea** (painful menstruation) and mittelschmerz (midcycle pain) without other organic pathology are seen frequently and may contribute to CPP in more than half of all cases.

4. **Chronic pelvic inflammatory disease** may cause CPP. Therefore, culturing for sexually transmitted agents should be a routine part of the evaluation.

Medical Diagnoses and Chronic Pelvic Pain	
Medical diagnosis/symptom source	**Prevalence**
Bowel dysmotility disorders	50 to 80%
Musculoskeletal disorders	30 to 70%
Cyclic gynecologic pain	20 to 50%
Urologic diagnoses	5 to 10%
Endometriosis, advanced and/or with dense bowel adhesions	Less than 5%
Unusual medical diagnoses	Less than 2%
Multiple medical diagnoses	30 to 50%
No identifiable medical diagnosis	Less than 5%

C. Nongynecologic medical problems

1. **Bowel dysmotility** (eg, irritable bowel syndrome and constipation) may be the primary symptom source in 50 percent of all cases of CPP and may be a contributing factor in up to 80 percent of cases. Pain from irritable bowel syndrome is typically described as a crampy, recurrent pain accompanied by abdominal distention and bloating, alternating diarrhea and constipation, and passage of mucus. The pain is often worse during or near the menstrual period. A highly suggestive sign is exquisite tenderness to palpation which improves with continued pressure.

2. **Musculoskeletal dysfunction,** including abdominal myofascial pain syndromes, can cause or contribute to CPP.

D. Psychologic problems

1. **Depressive disorders** contribute to more than half of all cases of CPP. Frequently, the pain becomes part of a cycle of pain, disability, and mood disturbance. The diagnostic criteria for depression include depressed mood, diminished interest in daily activities, weight loss or gain, insomnia or hypersomnia, psychomotor agitation or retardation,

fatigue, feelings of worthlessness, loss of concentration, and recurrent thoughts of death.

2. **Somatoform disorders,** including somatization disorder, contribute to 10 to 20 percent of cases of CPP. The essential feature of somatization disorder is a pattern of recurring, multiple, clinically significant somatic complaints.

II. Clinical evaluation of chronic pelvic pain

A. History

1. The character, intensity, distribution, and location of pain are important. Radiation of pain or should be assessed. The temporal pattern of the pain (onset, duration, changes, cyclicity) and aggravating or relieving factors (eg, posture, meals, bowel movements, voiding, menstruation, intercourse, medications) should be documented.

2. **Associated symptoms.** Anorexia, constipation, or fatigue are often present.

3. **Previous surgeries,** pelvic infections, infertility, or obstetric experiences may provide additional clues.

4. For patients of reproductive age, the timing and characteristics of their last menstrual period, the presence of non-menstrual vaginal bleeding or discharge, and the method of contraception used should be determined.

5. Life situations and events that affect the pain should be sought.

6. Gastrointestinal and urologic symptoms, including the relationship between these systems to the pain should be reviewed.

7. The patient's affect may suggest depression or other mood disorders.

B. Physical examination

1. If the woman indicates the location of her pain with a single finger, the pain is more likely caused by a discrete source than if she uses a sweeping motion of her hand.

2. A pelvic examination should be performed. Special attention should be given to the bladder, urethra.

3. The piriformis muscles should be palpated; piriformis spasm can cause pain when climbing stairs, driving a car, or when first arising in the morning. This muscle is responsible for external rotation of the hip and can be palpated posteriolaterally, cephalic to the ischial spine. This examination is most easily performed if the woman externally rotates her hip against the resistance of the examiner's other hand. Piriformis spasm is treated with physical therapy.

4. Abdominal deformity, erythema, edema, scars, hernias, or distension should be noted. Abnormal bowel sounds may suggest a gastrointestinal process.

5. Palpation should include the epigastrium, flanks, and low back, and inguinal areas.

C. Special tests

1. Initial laboratory tests should include cervical cytology, endocervical cultures for *Neisseria gonorrhoeae* and Chlamydia, stool hemoccult, and urinalysis. Other tests may be suggested by the history and examination.

2. Laparoscopy is helpful when the pelvic examination is abnormal or when initial therapy fails.

III. Management

A. Myofascial pain syndrome may be treated by a variety of physical therapy techniques. Trigger points can often be treated with injections of a local anesthetic (eg, bupivacaine [Marcaine]), with or without the addition of a corticosteroid.

B. If the pain is related to the menstrual cycle, treatment aimed at suppressing the cycle may help. Common methods to accomplish this include administration of depot medroxyprogesterone (Depo-Provera) and continuously dosed oral contraceptives.

C. Cognitive-behavioral therapy is appropriate for all women with CPP. Relaxation and distraction techniques are often helpful.

D. When endometriosis or pelvic adhesions are discovered on diagnostic laparoscopy, they are usually treated during the procedure. Hysterectomy may be warranted if the pain has persisted for more than six months, does not respond to analgesics (including anti-inflammatory agents), and impairs the woman's normal function.

E. **Antidepressants or sleeping aids** are useful adjunctive therapies. Amitriptyline (Elavil), in low doses of 25-50 mg qhs, may be of help in improving sleep and reducing the severity of chronic pain complaints.

F. **Muscle relaxants** may prove useful in patients with guarding, splinting, or reactive muscle spasms.

References: See page 140.

Endometriosis

Endometriosis is characterized by the presence of endometrial tissue on the ovaries, fallopian tubes or other abnormal sites, causing pain or infertility. Women are usually 25 to 29 years old at the time of diagnosis. Approximately 24 percent of women who complain of pelvic pain are subsequently found to have endometriosis. The overall prevalence of endometriosis is estimated to be 5 to 10 percent.

I. **Clinical evaluation**

A. Endometriosis should be considered in any woman of reproductive age who has pelvic pain. The most common symptoms are dysmenorrhea, dyspareunia, and low back pain that worsens during menses. Rectal pain and painful defecation may also occur. Other causes of secondary dysmenorrhea and chronic pelvic pain (eg, upper genital tract infections, adenomyosis, adhesions) may produce similar symptoms.

Differential Diagnosis of Endometriosis	

Generalized pelvic pain
Pelvic inflammatory disease
    Endometritis
    Pelvic adhesions
    Neoplasms, benign or
    malignant
    Ovarian torsion
    Sexual or physical abuse
    Nongynecologic causes
Dysmenorrhea
Primary
    Secondary (adenomyosis,
    myomas, infection, cervical
    stenosis)
	Dyspareunia
	Musculoskeletal causes (pelvic relaxation, levator spasm)
	Gastrointestinal tract (constipation, irritable bowel syndrome)
	Urinary tract (urethral syndrome, interstitial cystitis)
	Infection
	Pelvic vascular congestion
	Diminished lubrication or vaginal expansion because of insufficient arousal
	Infertility
	Male factor
	Tubal disease (infection)
	Anovulation
	Cervical factors (mucus, sperm antibodies, stenosis)
	Luteal phase deficiency

B. Infertility may be the presenting complaint for endometriosis. Infertile patients often have no painful symptoms.

C. **Physical examination.** The physician should palpate for a fixed, retroverted uterus, adnexal and uterine tenderness, pelvic masses or nodularity along the uterosacral ligaments. A rectovaginal examination should identify uterosacral, cul-de-sac or septal nodules. Most women with endometriosis have normal pelvic findings.

II. **Treatment**

A. Confirmatory laparoscopy is usually required before treatment is instituted. In women with few symptoms, an empiric trial of oral contraceptives or progestins may be warranted to assess pain relief.

B. Medical treatment

1. Initial therapy also should include a nonsteroidal anti-inflammatory drug.

    a. Naproxen (Naprosyn) 500 mg followed by 250 mg PO tid-qid prn [250, 375,500 mg].

    b. Naproxen sodium (Aleve) 200 mg PO tid prn.

    c. Naproxen sodium (Anaprox) 550 mg, followed by 275 mg PO tid-qid prn.

    d. Ibuprofen (Motrin) 800 mg, then 400 mg PO q4-6h prn.

    e. Mefenamic acid (Ponstel) 500 mg PO followed by 250 mg q6h prn.

2. **Progestational agents.** Progestins are similar to combination OCPs in their effects on FSH, LH and endometrial tissue. They may be associated with more bothersome adverse effects than OCPs. Progestins are effective in reducing the symptoms of endometriosis. Oral progestin regimens may include once-daily administration of medroxyprogesterone at the lowest effective dosage (5 to 20 mg). Depot medroxyprogesterone may be given intramuscularly every two weeks for two months at 100 mg per dose and then once a month for four months at 200 mg per dose.

3. **Oral contraceptive pills (OCPs)** suppress LH and FSH and prevent ovulation. Combination OCPs alleviate symptoms in about three quarters of patients. Oral contraceptives can be taken continuously (with no placebos) or cyclically, with a week of placebo pills between cycles. The OCPs can be discontinued after six months or continued indefinitely.

4. **Danazol (Danocrine)** has been highly effective in relieving the symptoms of endometriosis, but adverse effects may preclude its use. Adverse effects include headache, flushing, sweating and atrophic vaginitis. Androgenic side effects include acne, edema, hirsutism, deepening of the voice and weight gain. The initial dosage should be 800 mg per day, given in two divided oral doses. The overall response rate is 84 to 92 percent.

Medical Treatment of Endometriosis		
Drug	**Dosage**	**Adverse effects**
Danazol (Danocrine)	800 mg per day in 2 divided doses	Estrogen deficiency, androgenic side effects
Oral contraceptives	1 pill per day (continuous or cyclic)	Headache, nausea, hypertension
Medroxyproges-terone (Provera)	5 to 20 mg orally per day	Same as with other oral progestins
Medroxyproges-terone suspension (Depo-Provera)	100 mg IM every 2 weeks for 2 months; then 200 mg IM every month for 4 months or 150 mg IM every 3 months	Weight gain, depression, irregular menses or amenorrhea
Norethindrone (Aygestin)	5 mg per day orally for 2 weeks; then increase by 2.5 mg per day every 2 weeks up to 15 mg per day	Same as with other oral progestins
Leuprolide (Lupron)	3.75 mg IM every month for 6 months	Decrease in bone density, estrogen deficiency

Goserelin (Zoladex)	3.6 mg SC (in upper abdominal wall) every 28 days	Estrogen deficiency
Nafarelin (Synarel)	400 mg per day: 1 spray in 1 nostril in a.m.; 1 spray in other nostril in p.m.; start treatment on day 2 to 4 of menstrual cycle	Estrogen deficiency, bone density changes, nasal irritation

   C. **GnRH agonists.** These agents (eg, leuprolide [Lupron], goserelin
      [Zoladex]) inhibit the secretion of gonadotropin. GnRH agonists are
      contraindicated in pregnancy and have hypoestrogenic side effects. They
      produce a mild degree of bone loss. Because of concerns about
      osteopenia, "add-back" therapy with low-dose estrogen has been
      recommended. The dosage of leuprolide is a single monthly 3.75-mg
      depot injection given intramuscularly. Goserelin, in a dosage of 3.6 mg,
      is administered subcutaneously every 28 days. A nasal spray (nafarelin
      [Synarel]) may be used twice daily. The response rate is similar to that
      with danazol; about 90 percent of patients experience pain relief.
   D. **Surgical treatment**
      1. Surgical treatment is the preferred approach to infertile patients with
         advanced endometriosis. Laparoscopic ablation of endometriosis
         lesions may result in a 13 percent increase in the probability of
         pregnancy.
      2. Definitive surgery, which includes hysterectomy and oophorectomy,
         is reserved for women with intractable pain who no longer desire
         pregnancy.
References: See page 140.

Amenorrhea

Amenorrhea may be associated with infertility, endometrial hyperplasia, or
osteopenia. It may be the presenting sign of an underlying metabolic, endocrine,
congenital, or gynecologic disorder.

I. **Pathophysiology of amenorrhea**
   A. Amenorrhea may be caused by failure of the hypothalamic-pituitary-
      gonadal axis, by absence of end organs, or by obstruction of the outflow
      tract.
   B. **Menses** usually occur at intervals of 28 days, with a normal range of 18-
      40 days.
   C. **Amenorrhea** is defined as the absence of menstruation for 3 or more
      months in a women with past menses (secondary amenorrhea) or by the
      absence of menarche by age 16 in girls who have never menstruated
      (primary amenorrhea). Pregnancy is the most common cause of
      amenorrhea.
II. **Clinical evaluation of amenorrhea**
   A. **Menstrual history** should include the age of menarche, last menstrual
      period, and previous menstrual pattern. Diet, medications, and
      psychologic stress should be assessed.
   B. **Galactorrhea**, previous radiation therapy, chemotherapy, or recent weight
      gain or loss may provide important clues.
   C. **Prolonged, intense exercise**, often associated with dieting, can lead to
      amenorrhea. Symptoms of decreased estrogen include hot flushes and
      night sweats.
   D. **Physical examination**
      1. **Breast development and pubic hair distribution** should be assessed
         because they demonstrate exposure to estrogens and sexual maturity.
         Galactorrhea is a sign of hyperprolactinemia.
      2. **Thyroid gland** should be palpated for enlargement and nodules.

Abdominal striae in a nulliparous woman suggests hypercortisolism (Cushing's syndrome).
3. **Hair distribution** may reveal signs of androgen excess. The absence of both axillary and pubic hair in a phenotypically normal female suggests androgen insensitivity.
4. **External genitalia and vagina** should be inspected for atrophy from estrogen deficiency or clitoromegaly from androgen excess. An imperforate hymen or vaginal septum can block the outflow tract.
5. **Palpation of the uterus and ovaries** assures their presence and detects abnormalities.

III. **Diagnostic approach to amenorrhea**
   A. Menstrual flow requires an intact hypothalamic-pituitary-ovarian axis, a hormonally responsive uterus, and an intact outflow tract. The evaluation should localize the abnormality to either the uterus, ovary, anterior pituitary, or hypothalamus.
   B. **Step one--exclude pregnancy.** Pregnancy is the most common cause of secondary amenorrhea, and it must be excluded with a pregnancy test.
   C. **Step two--exclude hyperthyroidism and hyperprolactinemia**
      1. **Hypothyroidism and hyperprolactinemia** can cause amenorrhea. These disorders are excluded with a serum thyroid-stimulating hormone (TSH) and prolactin.
      2. **Hyperprolactinemia.** Prolactin inhibits the secretion of gonadotropin-releasing hormone. One-third of women with no obvious cause of amenorrhea have hyperprolactinemia. Mildly elevated prolactin levels should be confirmed by repeat testing and review the patient's medications. Hyperprolactinemia requires an MRI to exclude a pituitary tumor.

Drugs Associated with Amenorrhea	
Drugs that Increase Prolactin	Antipsychotics Tricyclic antidepressants Calcium channel blockers
Drugs with Estrogenic Activity	Digoxin, marijuana, oral contraceptives
Drugs with Ovarian Toxicity	Chemotherapeutic agents

   D. **Step three--assess estrogen status**
      1. **The progesterone challenge test** is used to determine estrogen status and determine the competence of the uterine outflow tract.
      2. Medroxyprogesterone (Provera) 10 mg is given PO qd for 10 consecutive days. Uterine bleeding within 2-7 days after completion is considered a positive test. A positive result suggests chronic anovulation, rather than hypothalamic-pituitary insufficiency or ovarian failure, and a positive test also confirms the presence of a competent outflow tract.
      3. A negative test indicates either an incompetent outflow tract, nonreactive endometrium, or inadequate estrogen stimulation.
         a. An abnormality of the outflow tract should be excluded with a regimen of conjugated estrogens (Premarin), 1.25 mg daily on days 1 through 21 of the cycle. Medroxyprogesterone (Provera) 10 mg is given on the last 5 days of the 21-day cycle. (A combination oral contraceptive agent can also be used.)
         b. Withdrawal bleeding within 2-7 days of the last dose of progesterone confirms the presence of an unobstructed outflow tract and a normal endometrium, and the problem is localized to the hypothalamic-pituitary axis or ovaries.
      4. In patients who have had prolonged amenorrhea, an endometrial biopsy should be considered before withdrawal bleeding is induced.

Biopsy can reveal endometrial hyperplasia.
  E. **Step four--evaluation of hypoestrogenic amenorrhea**
     1. Serum follicle-stimulating hormone (FSH) and luteinizing hormone (LH) levels should be measured to localize the problem to the ovary, pituitary or hypothalamus.
     2. **Ovarian failure**
        a. An FSH level greater than 50 mIU/mL indicates ovarian failure.
        b. Ovarian failure is considered "premature" when it occurs in women less than 40 years of age.
     3. **Pituitary or hypothalamic dysfunction**
        a. A normal or low gonadotropin level is indicative of pituitary or hypothalamic failure. An MRI is the most sensitive study to rule out a pituitary tumor.
        b. If MRI does not reveal a tumor, a defect in pulsatile GnRH release from the hypothalamus is the probable cause.
IV. **Management of chronic anovulation**
  A. Adequate estrogen and anovulation is indicated by withdrawal bleeding with the progesterone challenge test.
  B. Often there is a history of weight loss, psychosocial stress, or excessive exercise. Women usually have a normal or low body weight and normal secondary sex characteristics.
     1. Reducing stress and assuring adequate nutrition may induce ovulation. These women are at increased risk for endometrial cancer because of the hyperplastic effect of unopposed estrogen.
     2. Progesterone (10 mg/day for the first 7-10 days of every month) is given to induce withdrawal bleeding. If contraception is desired, a low-dose oral contraceptive should be used.
V. **Management of hypothalamic dysfunction**
  A. Amenorrheic women with a normal prolactin level, a negative progesterone challenge, with low or normal gonadotropin levels, and with a normal sella turcica imaging are considered to have hypothalamic dysfunction.
  B. Hypothalamic amenorrhea usually results from psychologic stress, depression, severe weight loss, anorexia nervosa, or strenuous exercise.
  C. Hypoestrogenic women are at risk for osteoporosis and cardiovascular disease. Oral contraceptives are appropriate in young women. Women not desiring contraception should take estrogen, 0.625 mg, with medroxyprogesterone (Provera) 2.5 mg, every day of the month. Calcium and vitamin D supplementation are also recommended.
VI. **Management of disorders of the outflow tract or uterus--intrauterine adhesions (Asherman syndrome)**
  A. Asherman syndrome is the most common outflow-tract abnormality that causes amenorrhea. This disorder should be considered if amenorrhea develops following curettage or endometritis.
  B. Hysterosalpingography will detect adhesions. Therapy consists of hysteroscopy and lysis of adhesions.
VII. **Management of disorders of the ovaries**
  A. Ovarian failure is suspected if menopausal symptoms are present. Women with premature ovarian failure who are less than 30 years of age should undergo karyotyping to rule out the presence of a Y chromosome. If a Y chromosome is detected, testicular tissue should be removed.
  B. Patients with ovarian failure should be prescribed estrogen 0.625 mg with progesterone 2.5 mg daily with calcium and vitamin D.
VIII. **Disorders of the anterior pituitary**
  A. Prolactin-secreting adenoma are excluded by MRI of the pituitary.
  B. Cabergoline (Dostinex) or bromocriptine (Parlodel) are used for most adenomas; surgery is considered later.
References: See page 140.

Menopause

The average age of menopause is 51 years, with a range of 41-55. Menopause occurs before age 40 in about 5% of women. Menopause is indicated by an elevated follicle-stimulating hormone (FSH) level greater than 40 mlU/mL.

I. **Pharmacologic therapy for symptoms of menopause**
  A. **Vasomotor instability.** A hot flush is a flushed or blushed feeling of the face, neck and upper chest. The most severe hot flushes usually occur at night. Estrogen therapy can reduce hot flushes.
  B. **Psychologic symptoms.** Mood swings, depression and concentration difficulties are associated with menopause. Estrogen improves mood or dysphoria associated with menopause.
  C. **Urogenital symptoms.** Declining estrogen levels lead to atrophy of the urogenital tissues and vaginal thinning and shortening, resulting in dyspareunia and urethral irritation. Urinary tract infections and urinary incontinence may develop. Estrogen treatment (oral or intravaginal) reduces these problems

II. **Pharmacologic management of long-term risks**
  A. **Coronary artery disease.** Physiologic effects of estrogen, such as arterial vasodilatation, increased high-density lipoprotein (HDL) cholesterol levels and decreased low-density lipoprotein (LDL) cholesterol levels, are likely to reduce cardiovascular risk.
  B. **Osteoporosis.** More than 250,000 hip fractures occur annually. Estrogen deficiency is the primary cause of osteoporosis, although many other secondary causes for osteoporosis exist (eg, poor diet, glucocorticoid excess). Thus, women at risk for osteoporosis should be considered candidates for HRT.

Minimum Effective Dosages of Estrogens for Prevention of Osteoporosis	
Formulation	**Minimum effective dosage**
Conjugated estrogen Premarin (0.3, 0.625, 0.9, 1.25, 2.5 mg)	0.625 mg
Micronized estradiol Estrace (0.5, 1.0, 2.0 mg)	1.0 mg

Esterified estrogen
  Estratab (0.3, 0.625, 2.5 mg)
  Menest (0.3, 0.625, 1.25, 2.5 mg)
	0.625 mg

Estropipate
  Ogen (0.625, 1.25, 2.5 mg)
  Ortho-Est (0.625, 1.25 mg)
	1.25 mg

Transdermal estradiol
  Climara (0.05, 0.1 mg)
  Estraderm (0.05, 0.1 mg)
	0.05 mg

Combination preparations	
Prempro	0.625 mg conjugated estrogen/2.5 mg or 5.0 mg medroxyprogesterone. Take one tab daily.
Premphase	0.625 mg conjugated estrogen (14 tablets) and 0.625 mg conjugated estrogen/5 mg medroxyprogesterone (14 tablets in sequence)
Combipatch	0.05 mg estradiol/0.14 mg norethindrone
Estratest	1.25 mg esterified estrogen/2.5 mg methyltestosterone
Estratest HS	0.625 mg esterified estrogen/1.25 mg methyltestosterone
Vaginal preparations	
Micronized estradiol cream (Estrace)	0.01% or 0.1 mg per g (42.5 g/tube)
Estropipate cream (Ogen)	1.5 mg per g (42.5 g/tube)
Conjugated estrogen cream (Premarin)	0.625 mg per g (42.5 g/tube)
Estradiol vaginal ring (Estring)	7.5 µg per 24 hours every 90 days

III. **Hormone replacement therapy administration and regimens**
   A. HRT should not be a universal recommendation. The benefits and risks associated with HRT must be weighed on an individual basis. A woman with significant risk factors for osteoporosis or CHD may benefit from long-term HRT. A woman with a personal or strong family history of breast cancer may not benefit from long-term HRT.
   B. Hormone users have a lower risk of death (relative risk, 0.63) than nonusers. This reduction is largest in women with cardiac risk factors. The benefit decreases with use of more than 10 years (due to breast cancer deaths) but still remains significant. HRT should increase life expectancy for nearly all women. The risk of HRT outweighs the benefit only in women without risk factors for CHD or hip fracture, but who have two first-degree relatives with breast cancer.
   C. Effective doses of estrogen for the prevention of osteoporosis are: 0.625 mg of conjugated estrogen, 0.5 mg of micronized estradiol, and 0.3 mg of esterified estrogen.
   D. In those women with a uterus, a progestin should be given continuously (2.5 mg of medroxyprogesterone per day) or in a sequential fashion [5-10 mg of medroxyprogesterone (Provera) for 12-14 days each month]. The most common HRT regimen consists of estrogen with or without progestin. The oral route of administration is preferable because of the

hepatic effect on HDL cholesterol levels.

Relative and Absolute Contraindications for Hormone Replacement Therapy	
Absolute contraindications	**Relative contraindications**
Estrogen-responsive breast cancer	Chronic liver disease
Endometrial cancer	Severe hypertriglyceridemia
Undiagnosed abnormal vaginal bleeding	Endometriosis
Active thromboembolic disease	Previous thromboembolic disease
History of malignant melanoma	Gallbladder disease

- E. **Estrogen cream**. 1/4 of an applicator(0.6 mg) daily for 1-2 weeks, then 2-3 times/week will usually relieve urogenital symptoms. This regimen is used concomitantly with oral estrogen.
- F. **Adverse effects** attributed to HRT include breast tenderness, breakthrough bleeding and thromboembolic disorders.
- G. **Bisphosphonates** inhibit osteoclast activity. Alendronate (Fosamax) is effective in increasing BMD and reducing fractures by 40 percent. Alendronate should be taken in an upright position with a full glass of water 30 minutes before eating to prevent esophagitis. Alendronate is indicated for osteoporosis in women who have a contraindication to estrogen.
- H. **Raloxifene (Evista)**, 60 mg qd, is a selective estrogen receptor modulator, FDA-labeled for prophylactic treatment of osteoporosis. This agent offers an alternative to traditional HRT. The modulator increases bone density (although only one-half as effectively as estrogen) and reduces total and LDL cholesterol levels.

IV. **Complementary therapies**
- A. **Adequate dietary calcium** intake is essential, and supplementation is helpful if dietary sources are inadequate. Total calcium intake should approximate 1,500 mg per day, which usually requires supplementation.
- B. **Vitamin D supplementation** (400 to 800 IU per day) is recommended for women who do not spend 30 minutes per day in the sun.
- C. **Treatment of low libido** consists of 1% testosterone gel (AndroGel). Testosterone gel is supplied in 2.5- or 5-gram packets that deliver 25 or 50 mg of testosterone to the skin surface. Start with ½ gm/day applied to the inner surface of a forearm daily and increase to 1 gm/day if necessary. Androgens are known to increase libido and protect bone mass.

References: See page 140.

Premenstrual Syndrome

Premenstrual syndrome (PMS) refers to a group of menstrually related disorders and symptoms that includes premenstrual dysphoric disorder (PDD) as well as affective disturbances, alterations in appetite, cognitive disturbance, fluid retention and various types of pain. Premenstrual symptoms affect up to 40 percent of women of reproductive age, with severe impairment occurring in 5 percent. PMS may have an onset at any time during the reproductive years and, once symptoms are established, they tend to remain fairly constant until menopause.

I. Clinical evaluation of premenstrual syndrome

Symptom Clusters Commonly Noted in Patients with PMS	
Affective Symptoms Depression or sadness Irritability Tension Anxiety Tearfulness or crying easily Restlessness or jitteriness Anger Loneliness Appetite change Food cravings Changes in sexual interest Pain Headache or migraine Back pain Breast pain Abdominal cramps General or muscular pain	**Cognitive or performance** Mood instability or mood swings Difficulty in concentrating Decreased efficiency Confusion Forgetfulness Accident-prone Social avoidance Temper outbursts Energetic **Fluid retention** Breast tenderness or swelling Weight gain Abdominal bloating or swelling Swelling of extremities **General somatic** Fatigue or tiredness Dizziness or vertigo Nausea Insomnia

II. Clinical evaluation of premenstrual syndrome

A. PMS involves an assortment of disabling physical and emotional symptoms that appear during the luteal phase and resolve within the first week of the follicular phase. Symptoms of PMS fall into four main categories: mood, somatic, cognitive, and behavioral.

B. No specific serum marker can be used to confirm the diagnosis. Premenstrual dysphoric disorder is diagnosed when mood symptoms predominate symptoms of PMS.

C. The differential diagnosis includes hypothyroidism, anemia, perimenopause, drug and alcohol abuse, and affective disorders. Common alternative diagnoses in patients complaining of PMS include affective or personality disorder, menopausal symptoms, eating disorder, and alcohol or other substance abuse. A medical condition such as diabetes or hypothyroidism, is the cause of the symptoms in 8.4%, and 10.6% have symptoms related to oral contraceptive (OC) use.

D. **Affective symptoms** of PMS strongly resemble major depression, except that PDD differs from major depression in that PDD occurs in the premenstrual phase alone. Selective serotonin reuptake inhibitors have been shown to be effective in the treatment of premenstrual dysphoria.

E. PMS is associated only with ovulatory menstrual cycles. While symptoms may occur with nonovulatory cycles, such as during therapy with oral contraceptives, the symptoms are believed to be hormonally related, because changing the contraceptive formulation usually alters the symptom pattern.

F. **Nutrient abnormalities.** Deficiencies of magnesium, manganese, B vitamins, vitamin E and linoleic acid and its metabolites have been reported in women with PMS. In addition, dietary deficiencies of calcium, magnesium and manganese have been described in women with menstrually related discomforts.

III. Primary treatment strategies

A. **Dietary modification.** The recommended dietary intake for the treatment of PMS consists of low-fat, low cholesterol, balanced diet.

B. **Nonsteroidal anti-inflammatory drugs**(NSAIDs) are effective for treatment of dysmenorrhea, and their use has been recommended for other perimenstrual discomforts.

C. **Antidepressants.** The lower side effect profile and efficacy data for the selective serotonin reuptake inhibitors support their use over other classes of antidepressants. Antidepressant therapy should be prescribed daily in the usual dosages for depression.

D. **Cognitive behavioral therapy.** Patients with expectations of negative symptoms or of impaired performance around menses may respond well to cognitive therapy.

E. **Hormonal contraceptives.** Combined oral contraceptive pills or a progestin-only contraceptive agent may provide relief of PMS.

F. **Diuretics.** Symptoms related to fluid retention can usually be eradicated through dietary measures, most specifically restriction of sodium and simple sugars. However, diuretics may be useful in patients with very troubling edema. Spironolactone has bee demonstrated to be effective in a dosage of 100 mg per day.

IV. **Treatments not generally recommended**

A. **Progesterone.** Multiple double-blind, placebo-controlled studies of progesterone have failed to show evidence of progesterone efficacy in PMS, and its use is not recommended.

B. **High-dose vitamin B6.** Controlled trials have failed to document its effectiveness. Peripheral neuropathy has been reported with daily dosages of 200 mg or more.

C. **Gonadotropin-Releasing Hormone Agonists or Antagonists.** The expense and side effect profile, including hypoestrogenism and an increase risk of osteoporosis, of these agents would recommend against their use for PMS.

DSM-IV Criteria for Premenstrual Dysphoric Disorder

- Five or more symptoms
- At least one of the following four symptoms:
    Markedly depressed mood, feelings of hopelessness, or self-deprecating thoughts
    Marked anxiety, tension, feeling of being "keyed up" or "on edge"
    Marked affective lability
    Persistent and marked anger or irritability or increase in interpersonal conflicts
- Additional symptoms that may be used to fulfill the criteria:
    Decreased interest in usual activities
    Subjective sense of difficulty in concentrating
    Lethargy, easy fatigability, or marked lack of energy
    Marked change in appetite, overeating, or specific food cravings
    Hypersomnia or insomnia
    Subjective sense of being overwhelmed or out of control
- Other physical symptoms such as breast tenderness or swelling, headaches, joint or muscle pain, a sensation of bloating, or weight gain
- Symptoms occurring during last week of luteal phase
- Symptoms are absent postmenstrually
- Disturbances that interfere with work or school or with usual social activities and relationships
- Disturbances that are not an exacerbation of symptoms of another disorder

---

V. **Treatment of premenstrual syndrome**

A. More than 70% of women with PMS will respond to therapy.

B. **Symptomatic treatment**

1. **Fluid retention and bloating** may be relieved by limiting salty foods. If 5 pounds or more are gained during the luteal phase, diuretic therapy may be effective. Spironolactone (Aldactone) is the drug of choice because of its potassium-sparing effects. The dose ranges from 25-200 mg qd during the luteal phase.

2. **Mastalgia.** Support bras, decreased caffeine intake, nutritional supplements (vitamin E, 400 IU), a low-fat diet, oral contraceptives, or non-steroidal anti-inflammatory drugs (NSAIDs) are effective. Cabergoline (Dostinex), 0.25 mg - 1 mg twice a week during the luteal phase may be effective. Side effects include dizziness and gastrointestinal upset.
3. **Sleep disturbances.** Conservative measures include regulating sleep patterns, avoiding stimulating events before bedtime, and progressive relaxation and biofeedback therapy. Doxepin (Sinequan), 10-25 mg hs, also is effective.

Treatment of Premenstrual Syndrome

Fluoxetine (Prozac) 5-20 mg qd
Sertraline (Zoloft) 25-50 mg qd
Paroxetine (Paxil) 5-20 mg qd
Buspirone (BuSpar) 25 mg qd in divided doses

Alprazolam (Xanax) 0.25-0.50 mg tid

Mefenamic acid (Ponstel) 250 mg tid with meals
Oral contraceptives

Calcium, 600 mg bid, may help decrease negative mood, fluid retention, and pain
Magnesium 100 mg qd may help decrease negative mood, fluid retention, and pain
Manganese 400 mg qd
Vitamin E, 400 IU qd

Other
Cabergoline (Dostinex) 0.25 mg - 1 mg twice a week during the luteal phase for breast pain
Spirolactone (Aldactone) 25-200 mg qd

---

4. **Menstrual migraines** often occur just before and during menses. Menstrual migraines are treated with NSAIDs, sumatriptan (Imitrex), 50 mg po or 30-60 mg intramuscularly (IM) or propranolol (Inderal), 80-240 mg in divided doses; or amitriptyline (Elavil), 25-100 mg, taken before bedtime.

VI. **Syndromal treatment**
   A. Nonpharmacologic remedies include calcium (600 mg bid) and magnesium (360 mg qd), possibly with the addition of vitamins.
   B. SSRIs are appropriate for women with mood symptoms. Administration of fluoxetine (Prozac), 20 mg, or sertraline (Zoloft), 25-50 mg, has shown efficacy.

Lifestyle Modifications That Help Relieve Premenstrual Syndrome

Moderate, regular, aerobic exercise (1-2 miles of brisk walking 4-5 times/week) may decrease depression and pain symptoms

Reducing or eliminating salt and alcohol, especially in the luteal phase; eating small, frequent meals; increasing complex carbohydrates

---

   C. **Anxiolytics and antidepressants. Alprazolam (Xanax),** 0.25-0.5 mg tid, given during the luteal phase only may relieve anxiety.
   D. **Surgery.** Oophorectomy is reserved for patients whose symptoms have resolved completely for 4-6 months with GnRH agonists, who have completed child bearing, and who require more than 5 years of long-term suppression.

References: See page 140.

Abnormal Vaginal Bleeding

Menorrhagia (excessive bleeding) is most commonly caused by anovulatory menstrual cycles. Occasionally it is caused by thyroid dysfunction, infections or cancer.

I. **Pathophysiology of normal menstruation**
   A. In response to gonadotropin-releasing hormone from the hypothalamus, the pituitary gland synthesizes follicle-stimulating hormone (FSH) and luteinizing hormone (LH), which induce the ovaries to produce estrogen and progesterone.
   B. During the follicular phase, estrogen stimulation causes an increase in endometrial thickness. After ovulation, progesterone causes endometrial maturation. Menstruation is caused by estrogen and progesterone withdrawal.
   C. **Abnormal bleeding** is defined as bleeding that occurs at intervals of less than 21 days, more than 36 days, lasting longer than 7 days, or blood loss greater than 80 mL.

II. **Clinical evaluation of abnormal vaginal bleeding**
   A. A menstrual and reproductive history should include last menstrual period, regularity, duration, frequency; the number of pads used per day, and intermenstrual bleeding.
   B. Stress, exercise, weight changes and systemic diseases, particularly thyroid, renal or hepatic diseases or coagulopathies, should be sought. The method of birth control should be determined.
   C. Pregnancy complications, such as spontaneous abortion, ectopic pregnancy, placenta previa and abruptio placentae, can cause heavy bleeding. Pregnancy should always be considered as a possible cause of abnormal vaginal bleeding.

III. **Puberty and adolescence--menarche to age 16**
   A. Irregularity is normal during the first few months of menstruation; however, soaking more than 25 pads or 30 tampons during a menstrual period is abnormal.
   B. Absence of premenstrual symptoms (breast tenderness, bloating, cramping) is associated with anovulatory cycles.
   C. Fever, particularly in association with pelvic or abdominal pain may, indicate pelvic inflammatory disease. A history of easy bruising suggests a coagulation defect. Headaches and visual changes suggest a pituitary tumor.
   D. **Physical findings**
      1. Pallor not associated with tachycardia or signs of hypovolemia suggests chronic excessive blood loss secondary to anovulatory bleeding, adenomyosis, uterine myomas, or blood dyscrasia.
      2. Fever, leukocytosis, and pelvic tenderness suggests PID.
      3. Signs of impending shock indicate that the blood loss is related to pregnancy (including ectopic), trauma, sepsis, or neoplasia.
      4. Pelvic masses may represent pregnancy, uterine or ovarian neoplasia, or a pelvic abscess or hematoma.
      5. Fine, thinning hair, and hypoactive reflexes suggest hypothyroidism.
      6. Ecchymoses or multiple bruises may indicate trauma, coagulation defects, medication use, or dietary extremes.
   E. **Laboratory tests**
      1. CBC and platelet count and a urine or serum pregnancy test should be obtained.
      2. Screening for sexually transmitted diseases, thyroid function, and coagulation disorders (partial thromboplastin time, INR, bleeding time) should be completed.
      3. **Endometrial sampling** is rarely necessary for those under age 20.
   F. **Treatment of infrequent bleeding**
      1. Therapy should be directed at the underlying cause when possible. If

the CBC and other initial laboratory tests are normal and the history and physical examination are normal, reassurance is usually all that is necessary.

2. Ferrous gluconate, 325 mg bid-tid, should be prescribed.

G. Treatment of frequent or heavy bleeding

1. Treatment with nonsteroidal anti-inflammatory drugs (NSAIDs) improves platelet aggregation and increases uterine vasoconstriction. NSAIDs are the first choice in the treatment of menorrhagia because they are well tolerated and do not have the hormonal effects of oral contraceptives.

   a. Mefenamic acid (Ponstel) 500 mg tid during the menstrual period.

   b. Naproxen (Anaprox, Naprosyn) 500 mg loading dose, then 250 mg tid during the menstrual period.

   c. Ibuprofen (Motrin, Nuprin) 400 mg tid during the menstrual period.

   d. Gastrointestinal distress is common. NSAIDs are contraindicated in renal failure and peptic ulcer disease.

2. Iron should also be added as ferrous gluconate 325 mg tid.

H. Patients with hypovolemia or a hemoglobin level below 7 g/dL should be hospitalized for hormonal therapy and iron replacement.

1. Hormonal therapy consists of estrogen (Premarin) 25 mg IV q6h until bleeding stops. Thereafter, oral contraceptive pills should be administered q6h x 7 days, then taper slowly to one pill qd.

2. If bleeding continues, IV vasopressin (DDAVP) should be administered. Hysteroscopy may be necessary, and dilation and curettage is a last resort. Transfusion may be indicated in severe hemorrhage.

3. Iron should also be added as ferrous gluconate 325 mg tid.

IV. **Primary childbearing years--ages 16 to early 40s**

A. Contraceptive complications and pregnancy are the most common causes of abnormal bleeding in this age group. Anovulation accounts for 20% of cases.

B. Adenomyosis, endometriosis, and fibroids increase in frequency as a woman ages, as do endometrial hyperplasia and endometrial polyps. Pelvic inflammatory disease and endocrine dysfunction may also occur.

C. **Laboratory tests**

1. CBC and platelet count, Pap smear, and pregnancy test.

2. Screening for sexually transmitted diseases, thyroid-stimulating hormone, and coagulation disorders (partial thromboplastin time, INR, bleeding time).

3. If a non-pregnant woman has a pelvic mass, ultrasonography or hysterosonography (with uterine saline infusion) is required.

D. **Endometrial sampling**

1. Long-term unopposed estrogen stimulation in anovulatory patients can result in endometrial hyperplasia, which can progress to adenocarcinoma; therefore, in perimenopausal patients who have been anovulatory for an extended interval, the endometrium should be biopsied.

2. Biopsy is also recommended before initiation of hormonal therapy for women over age 30 and for those over age 20 who have had prolonged bleeding.

3. Hysteroscopy and endometrial biopsy with a Pipelle aspirator should be done on the first day of menstruation (to avoid an unexpected pregnancy) or anytime if bleeding is continuous.

E. **Treatment**

1. Medical protocols for anovulatory bleeding (dysfunctional uterine bleeding) are similar to those described above for adolescents.

2. **Hormonal therapy**

   a. In women who do not desire immediate fertility, hormonal therapy may be used to treat menorrhagia.

   b. A 21-day package of oral contraceptives is used. The patient should take one pill three times a day for 7 days. During the 7 days of therapy, bleeding should subside, and, following treatment, heavy flow will occur. After 7 days off the hormones, another 21-day package is initiated, taking one pill each day for 21 days, then no pills for 7 days.

    c. Alternatively, medroxyprogesterone (Provera), 10-20 mg per day for days 16 through 25 of each month, will result in a reduction of menstrual blood loss. Pregnancy will not be prevented.

    d. Patients with severe bleeding may have hypotension and tachycardia. These patients require hospitalization, and estrogen (Premarin) should be administered IV as 25 mg q4-6h until bleeding slows (up to a maximum of four doses). Oral contraceptives should be initiated concurrently as described above.

3. Iron should also be added as ferrous gluconate 325 mg tid.

4. Surgical treatment can be considered if childbearing is completed and medical management fails to provide relief.

V. Premenopausal, perimenopausal, and postmenopausal years--age 40 and over

A. Anovulatory bleeding accounts for about 90% of abnormal vaginal bleeding in this age group. However, bleeding should be considered to be from cancer until proven otherwise.

B. History, physical examination and laboratory testing are indicated as described above. Menopausal symptoms, personal or family history of malignancy and use of estrogen should be sought. A pelvic mass requires an evaluation with ultrasonography.

C. Endometrial carcinoma

1. In a perimenopausal or postmenopausal woman, amenorrhea preceding abnormal bleeding suggests endometrial cancer. Endometrial evaluation is necessary before treatment of abnormal vaginal bleeding.

2. Before endometrial sampling, determination of endometrial thickness by transvaginal ultrasonography is useful because biopsy is often not required when the endometrium is less than 5 mm thick.

D. Treatment

1. Cystic hyperplasia or endometrial hyperplasia without cytologic atypia is treated with depo-medroxyprogesterone, 200 mg IM, then 100 to 200 mg IM every 3 to 4 weeks for 6 to 12 months. Endometrial hyperplasia requires repeat endometrial biopsy every 3 to 6 months.

2. Atypical hyperplasia requires fractional dilation and curettage, followed by progestin therapy or hysterectomy.

3. If the patient's endometrium is normal (or atrophic) and contraception is a concern, a low-dose oral contraceptive may be used. If contraception is not needed, estrogen and progesterone therapy should be prescribed.

4. **Surgical management**

    a. **Vaginal or abdominal hysterectomy** is the most absolute curative treatment.

    b. **Dilatation and curettage** can be used as a temporizing measure to stop bleeding.

    c. **Endometrial ablation and resection** by laser, electrodiathermy "rollerball," or excisional resection are alternatives to hysterectomy.

References: See page 140.

Breast Cancer Screening

Breast cancer is the most common form of cancer in women. There are 200,000 new cases of breast cancer each year, resulting in 47,000 deaths per year. The lifetime risk of breast cancer is one in eight for a woman who is age 20. For patients under age 60, the chance of being diagnosed with breast cancer is 1 in about 400 in a given year.

I. Pathophysiology

A. The etiology of breast cancer remains unknown, but two breast cancer

genes have been cloned–the BRCA-1 and the BRCA-2 genes. Only 10% of all of the breast cancers can be explained by mutations in these genes.
   B. Estrogen stimulation is an important promoter of breast cancer, and, therefore, patients who have a long history of menstruation are at increased risk. Early menarche and late menopause are risk factors for breast cancer. Late age at birth of first child or nulliparity also increase the risk of breast cancer.
   C. Family history of breast cancer in a first degree relative and history of benign breast disease also increase the risk of breast cancer. The use of estrogen replacement therapy or oral contraceptives slightly increases the risk of breast cancer. Radiation exposure and alcoholic beverage consumption also increase the risk of breast cancer.

Recommended Intervals for Breast Cancer Screening Studies			
	Age <40 yr	**40-49 yr**	**50-75 yr**
Breast Self-Examination	Monthly by age 30	Monthly	Monthly
Professional Breast Examination	Every 3 yr, ages 20-39	Annually	Annually
Mammography, Low Risk Patient		Annually	Annually
Mammography, High Risk Patient	Begin at 35 yr	Annually	Annually

II. **Diagnosis and evaluation**
   A. **Clinical evaluation of a breast mass** should assess duration of the lesion, associated pain, relationship to the menstrual cycle or exogenous hormone use, and change in size since discovery. The presence of nipple discharge and its character (bloody or tea-colored, unilateral or bilateral, spontaneous or expressed) should be assessed.
   B. **Menstrual history.** The date of last menstrual period, age of menarche, age of menopause or surgical removal of the ovaries, regularity of the menstrual cycle, previous pregnancies, age at first pregnancy, and lactation history should be determined.
   C. **History of previous breast biopsies,** breast cancer, or cyst aspiration should be investigated. Previous or current oral contraceptive and hormone replacement therapy and dates and results of previous mammograms should be ascertained.
   D. **Family history** should document breast cancer in relatives and the age at which family members were diagnosed.
III. **Physical examination**
   A. The breasts should be inspected for asymmetry, deformity, skin retraction, erythema, peau d'orange (indicating breast edema), and nipple retraction, discoloration, or inversion.
   B. **Palpation**
      1. The breasts should be palpated while the patient is sitting and then supine with the ipsilateral arm extended. The entire breast should be palpated systematically.
      2. The mass should be evaluated for size, shape, texture, tenderness, fixation to skin or chest wall. The location of the mass should be documented with a diagram in the patient's chart. The nipples should be expressed to determine whether discharge can be induced. Nipple discharge should be evaluated for single or multiple ducts, color, and any associated mass.

3. The axillae should be palpated for adenopathy, with an assessment of size of the lymph nodes, their number, and fixation. The supraclavicular and cervical nodes should also be assessed.

IV. **Breast imaging**
  A. **Mammography**
    1. **Screening mammography** is performed in the asymptomatic patients and consists of two views. Patients are not examined by a mammographer. Screening mammography reduces mortality from breast cancer and should usually be initiated at age 40.
    2. **Diagnostic mammography** is performed after a breast mass has been detected. Patients usually are examined by a mammographer, and films are interpreted immediately and additional views of the lesion are completed. Mammographic findings predictive of malignancy include spiculated masses with architectural distortion and microcalcifications. A normal mammography in the presence of a palpable mass does not exclude malignancy.
  B. **Ultrasonography** is used as an adjunct to mammography to differentiate solid from cystic masses. It is the primary imaging modality in patients younger than 30 years old.

V. **Methods of breast biopsy**
  A. **Stereotactic core needle biopsy**. Using a computer-driven stereotactic unit, the lesion is localized in three dimensions, and an automated biopsy needle obtains samples. The sensitivity and specificity of this technique are 95-100% and 94-98%, respectively.
  B. **Palpable masses. Fine-needle aspiration biopsy (FNAB)** has a sensitivity ranging from 90-98%. Nondiagnostic aspirates require surgical biopsy.
    1. The skin is prepped with alcohol and the lesion is immobilized with the nonoperating hand. A 10 mL syringe, with a 18 to 22 gauge needle, is introduced in to the central portion of the mass at a 90° angle. When the needle enters the mass, suction is applied by retracting the plunger, and the needle is advanced. The needle is directed into different areas of the mass while maintaining suction on the syringe.
    2. Suction is slowly released before the needle is withdrawn from the mass. The contents of the needle are placed onto glass slides for pathologic examination.
  C. **Impalpable lesions**
    1. **Needle localized biopsy**
      a. Under mammographic guidance, a needle and hookwire are placed into the breast parenchyma adjacent to the lesion. The patient is taken to the operating room along with mammograms for an excisional breast biopsy.
      b. The skin and underlying tissues are infiltrated with 1% lidocaine with epinephrine. For lesions located within 5 cm of the nipple, a periareolar incision may be used or use a curved incision located over the mass and parallel to the areola. Incise the skin and subcutaneous fat, then palpate the lesion and excise the mass.
      c. After removal of the specimen, a specimen x-ray is performed to confirm that the lesion has been removed. The specimen can then be sent fresh for pathologic analysis.
      d. Close the subcutaneous tissues with a 4-0 chromic catgut suture, and close the skin with 4-0 subcuticular suture.

References: See page 140.

Breast Disorders

I. Nipple Discharge
A. Clinical evaluation
1. Nipple discharge may be a sign of cancer; therefore, it must be thoroughly evaluated. About 8% of biopsies performed for nipple discharge demonstrate cancer. The duration, bilaterality or unilaterality of the discharge, and the presence of blood should be determined. A history of oral contraceptives, hormone preparations, phenothiazines, nipple or breast stimulation or lactation should be sought. Discharges that flow spontaneously are more likely to be pathologic to discharges that must be manually expressed.
2. Unilateral, pink colored, bloody or non-milky discharge, or discharges associated with a mass are the discharges of most concern. Milky discharge can be caused by oral contraceptive agents, estrogen replacement therapy, phenothiazines, prolactinoma, or hypothyroidism. Nipple discharge secondary to malignancy is more likely to occur in older patients.
3. **Risk factors.** The assessment should identify risk factors, including age over 50 years, past personal history of breast cancer, history of hyperplasia on previous breast biopsies, and family history of breast cancer in a first-degree relative (mother, sister, daughter).

B. Physical examination
should include inspection of the breast for ulceration or contour changes and inspection of the nipple. Palpation should be performed with the patient in both the upright and the supine positions to determine the presence of a mass.

C. Diagnostic evaluation
1. **Bloody discharge.** A mammogram of the involved breast should be obtained if the patient is over 35 years old and has not had a mammogram within the preceding 6 months. Biopsy of any suspicious lesions should be completed.
2. **Watery, unilateral discharge** should be referred to a surgeon for evaluation and possible biopsy.
3. **Non-bloody discharge** should be tested for the presence of blood with a Hemoccult card. Nipple discharge secondary to carcinoma usually contains hemoglobin.
4. **Milky, bilateral discharge** should be evaluated with assays of prolactin and thyroid stimulating hormone to exclude an endocrinologic cause.
   a. A mammogram should also be performed if the patient is due for routine mammographic screening.
   b. If results of the mammogram and the endocrinologic screening studies are normal, the patient should return for a follow-up visit in 6 months to ensure that there has been no specific change in the character of the discharge, such as development of bleeding.

II. Breast Pain
A.
Determine the duration and location of the pain, associated trauma, previous breast surgery, associated lumps, or nipple discharge.
B.
Pain is an uncommon presenting symptom for breast cancer; however, cancer must be excluded. Cancer is the etiology in 5% of patients with breast pain. Pain that is associated with breast cancer is usually unilateral, intense, and constant.
C. Patients less than 35 years of age without a mass
1. Pain is unlikely to be a symptom of cancer.
2. A follow-up clinical breast examination should be performed in 1-2 months. Diagnostic mammography is usually not helpful but may be considered.
D. Patients 35 years of age or older
1. Obtain diagnostic mammogram, and obtain an ultrasound if a cystic lesion is present.
2. If studies are negative, a follow-up examination in 1-2 months is appropriate. If a suspicious lesion is detected, biopsy is required.

E. **Mastodynia**
  1. Mastodynia is defined as breast pain in the absence of a mass or other pathologic abnormality.
  2. **Causes of mastodynia** include menstrually related pain, costochondritis, trauma, and sclerosing adenosis.

III. **Fibrocystic Complex**
  A. Breast changes are usually multifocal, bilateral, and diffuse. One or more isolated fibrocystic lumps or areas of asymmetry may be present. The areas are usually tender.
  B. This disorder predominantly occurs in women with premenstrual abnormalities, nulliparous women, and nonusers of oral contraceptives.
  C. The disorder usually begins in mid-20's or early 30's. Tenderness is associated with menses and lasts about a week. The upper outer quadrant of the breast is most frequently involved bilaterally. There is no increased risk of cancer for the majority of patients.
  D. Suspicious areas may be evaluated by fine needle aspiration (FNA) cytology. If mammography and FNA are negative for cancer, and the clinical examination is benign, open biopsy is generally not needed.
  E. **Medical management of fibrocystic complex**
    1. **Oral contraceptives** are effective for severe breast pain in most young women. Start with a pill that contains low amounts of estrogen and relatively high amounts of progesterone (Loestrin, LoOvral, Ortho-Cept).
    2. If oral contraceptives do not provide relief, medroxyprogesterone, 5-10 mg/day from days 15-25 of each cycle, is added.
    3. A professionally fitted support bra often provides significant relief.
    4. A low fat diet, vitamins (E and B complex), evening primrose oil, and stopping smoking may provide relief.
    5. NSAIDs and cabergoline (Dostinex) may also be used.

References: See page 140.

Sexual Assault

Sexual assault is defined as any sexual act performed by one person on another without the person's consent. Sexual assault includes genital, anal, or oral penetration by a part of the accused's body or by an object. It may result from force, the threat of force, or the victim's inability to give consent. The annual incidence of sexual assault is 200 per 100,000 persons, accounting for 6% of all violent crimes. Approximately one in five women is sexually assaulted by the time she is 21 years of age.

I. **Psychologic effects**
  A. A woman who is sexually assaulted loses control over her life during the period of the assault. Her integrity and her life are threatened. She may experience intense anxiety, anger, or fear. After the assault, a "rape-trauma" syndrome often occurs. The immediate response may last for hours or days and is characterized by generalized pain, headache, chronic pelvic pain, eating and sleep disturbances, vaginal symptoms, depression, anxiety, and mood swings.
  B. The delayed phase is characterized by flashbacks, nightmares, and phobias.

II. **Medical evaluation**
  A. Informed consent must be obtained before the examination. Acute injuries should be stabilized. About 1% of injuries require hospitalization and major operative repair, and 0.1% of injuries are fatal.
  B. A history and physical examination should be performed. A chaperon should be present during the history and physical examination to reassure the victim and provide support. The patient should be asked to state in her own words what happened, identify her attacker if possible, and provide details of the act(s) performed if possible.

Clinical Care of the Sexual Assault Victim

Medical
Obtain informed consent from the patient
Obtain a gynecologic history
Assess and treat physical injuries
Obtain appropriate cultures and treat any existing infections
Provide prophylactic antibiotic therapy and offer immunizations
Provide therapy to prevent unwanted conception
Offer baseline serologic tests for hepatitis B virus, human immunodeficiency virus (HIV), and syphilis
Provide counseling
Arrange for follow-up medical care and counseling

Legal
Provide accurate recording of events
Document injuries
Collect samples (pubic hair, fingernail scrapings, vaginal secretions, saliva, blood-stained clothing)
Report to authorities as required
Assure chain of evidence

C. Previous obstetric and gynecologic conditions should be sought, particularly infections, pregnancy, use of contraception, and date of the last menstrual period. Preexisting pregnancy, risk for pregnancy, and the possibility of preexisting infections should be assessed.

D. **Physical examination** of the entire body and photographs or drawings of the injured areas should be completed. Bruises, abrasions, and lacerations should be sought. Superficial or extensive lacerations of the hymen and vagina, injury to the urethra, and occasionally rupture of the vaginal vault into the abdominal cavity may be noted. Bite marks are common.
   1. **Pelvic examination** should assess the status of the reproductive organs, collect samples from the cervix and vagina, and test for Neisseria gonorrhoeae and Chlamydia trachomatis.
   2. **A Wood light** should be used to find semen on the patient's body: dried semen will fluoresce. Sperm and other Y-chromosome-bearing cells may be identified from materials collected from victims.

E. **A serum sample** should be obtained for baseline serology for syphilis, herpes simplex virus, hepatitis B virus, and HIV.

F. **Trichomonas** is the most frequently acquired STD. The risk of acquiring human immunodeficiency virus (HIV) <1% during a single act of heterosexual intercourse, but the risk depends on the population involved and the sexual acts performed. The risk of acquiring gonorrhea is 6–12%, and the risk of acquiring syphilis is 3%.

G. **Hepatitis B virus** is 20 times more infectious than HIV during sexual intercourse. Hepatitis B immune globulin (0.06 mL of hepatitis B immune globulin per kilogram) should be administered intramuscularly as soon as possible within 14 days of exposure. It is followed by the standard three-dose immunization series with hepatitis B vaccine (0, 1, and 6 months), beginning at the time of hepatitis B immune globulin administration.

H. **Emergency contraception.** If the patient is found to be at risk for pregnancy as a result of the assault, emergency contraception should be offered. The risk of pregnancy after sexual assault is 2–4% in victims not already using contraception. One dose of combination oral contraceptive tablets is given at the time the victim is seen and an additional dose is given in 12 hours. Emergency contraception can be effective up to 120 hours after unprotected coitus. Metoclopramide (Reglan), 20 mg with each dose of hormone, is prescribed for nausea. A pregnancy test should be performed at the 2-week return visit if conception is suspected.

Emergency Contraception

1. Consider pretreatment one hour before each oral contraceptive pill dose, using one of the following orally administered antiemetic agents:
   Prochlorperazine (Compazine), 5 to 10 mg
   Promethazine (Phenergan), 12.5 to 25 mg
   Trimethobenzamide (Tigan), 250 mg
2. Administer the first dose of oral contraceptive pill within 72 hours of intercourse, and administer the second dose 12 hours after the first dose. Brand name options for emergency contraception include the following:
   Preven Kit--two pills per dose (0.5 mg of levonorgestrel and 100 μg of ethinyl estradiol per dose) Ovral--two pills per dose (0.5 mg of levonorgestrel and 100 μg of ethinyl estradiol per dose)
   Nordette--four pills per dose (0.6 mg of levonorgestrel and 120 μg of ethinyl estradiol per dose)
   Triphasil--four pills per dose (0.5 mg of levonorgestrel and 120 μg of ethinyl estradiol per dose)
   Plan B--one pill per dose (0.75 mg of levonorgestrel per dose)

Screening and Treatment of Sexually Transmissible Infections Following Sexual Assault

Initial Examination

Infection
- Testing for and gonorrhea and chlamydia from specimens from any sites of penetration or attempted penetration
- Wet mount and culture or a vaginal swab specimen for Trichomonas
- Serum sample for syphilis, herpes simplex virus, hepatitis B virus, and HIV

Pregnancy Prevention

Prophylaxis
- Hepatitis B virus vaccination and hepatitis B immune globulin.
- Empiric recommended antimicrobial therapy for chlamydial, gonococcal, and trichomonal infections and for bacterial vaginosis:
  Ceftriaxone, 125 mg intramuscularly in a single dose, plus
  Metronidazole, 2 g orally in a single dose, plus
  Doxycycline 100 mg orally two times a day for 7 days
  Azithromycin (Zithromax) is used if the patient is unlikely to comply with the 7 day course of doxycycline; single dose of four 250 mg caps.
  If the patient is penicillin-allergic, ciprofloxacin 500 mg PO or ofloxacin 400 mg PO is substituted for ceftriaxone. If the patient is pregnant, erythromycin 500 mg PO qid for 7 days is substituted for doxycycline.
  HIV prophylaxis consists of zidovudine (AZT) 200 mg PO tid, plus lamivudine (3TC) 150 mg PO bid for 4 weeks.

Follow-Up Examination (2 weeks)

- Cultures for N gonorrhoeae and C trachomatis (not needed if prophylactic treatment has been provided)
- Wet mount and culture for T vaginalis
- Collection of serum sample for subsequent serologic analysis if test results are positive

---

Follow-Up Examination (12 weeks)

Serologic tests for infectious agents:
   T pallidum
   HIV (repeat test at 6 months)
   Hepatitis B virus (not needed if hepatitis B virus vaccine was given)

III. **Emotional care**
   A. The physician should discuss the injuries and the probability of infection or pregnancy with the victim, and she should be allowed to express her anxieties.
   B. Anxiolytic medication may be useful; lorazepam (Ativan) 1-5 mg PO tid prn anxiety.
   C. The patient should be referred to personnel trained to handle rape-trauma victims within 1 week.

IV. **Follow-up care**
   A. The patient is seen for medical follow-up in 2 weeks for documentation of healing of injuries.
   B. Repeat testing includes syphilis, hepatitis B, and gonorrhea and chlamydia cultures. HIV serology should be repeated in 3 months and 6 months.
   C. A pregnancy test should be performed if conception is suspected.

References: See page 140.

Osteoporosis

Osteoporosis is a common cause of skeletal fractures. Bone loss accelerates during menopause due to a decrease in estrogen production. Approximately 20% of women have osteoporosis in their seventh decade of life, 30% of women in their eighth decade of life, and 70% of women older than 80 years.

I. **Diagnosis**
   A. **Risk factors** for osteoporosis include female gender, increasing age, family history, Caucasian or Asian race, estrogen deficient state, nulliparity, sedentarism, low calcium intake, smoking, excessive alcohol or caffeine consumption, and use of glucocorticoid drugs. Patients who have already sustained a fracture have a markedly increased risk of sustaining further fractures.
   B. **Bone density testing.** Bone density is the strongest predictor of fracture risk. Bone density can be assessed by dual X-ray absorptiometry.

Indications for Bone Density Testing

Estrogen-deficient women at clinical risk for osteoporosis
Individuals with vertebral abnormalities
Individuals receiving, or planning to receive, long-term glucocorticoid therapy
Individuals with primary hyperparathyroidism
Individuals being monitored to assess the response of an osteoporosis drug

---

II. **Prevention and treatment strategies**
   A. A balanced diet including 1000-1500 mg of calcium, weight bearing exercise, and avoidance of alcohol and tobacco products should be encouraged. Daily calcium supplementation (1000-1500 mg) along with 400-800 IU vitamin D should be recommended.
   B. Estrogen therapy is recommended for most females. Females who are not willing or incapable of receiving estrogen therapy and have osteopenic bone densities may consider alendronate and raloxifene. After the age of 65, a bone density test should be performed to decide if pharmacologic

therapy should be considered to prevent or treat osteoporosis.

Drugs for Osteoporosis

Drug	Dosage	Indication	Comments
Estrogen	0.625 mg qd with medroxyprogesterone (Provera), 2.5 mg qd	Prevention and Treatment	Recommended for most menopausal females
Raloxifene (Evista)	60 mg PO QD	Prevention	No breast or uterine tissue stimulation. Decrease in cholesterol similar to estrogen.
Alendronate (Fosamax)	5 mg PO QD 10 mg PO QD	Prevention Treatment	Take in the morning with 2-3 glasses of water, at least 30 min before any food, beverages, or medication. Reduction in fracture risk.
Calcitonin	200 IU QD (nasal) 50-100 IU QD SQ	Treatment	Modest analgesic effect. Not indicated in the early post-menopausal years.
Calcium	1000-1500 mg/day	Prevention/ Treatment	Calcium alone may not prevent osteoporosis
Vitamin D	400-800 IU QD	Prevention/ Treatment	May help reduce hip fracture incidence

C. Estrogen replacement therapy
   1. Postmenopausal women without contraindications should consider ERT. Contraindications include a family or individual history of breast cancer; estrogen dependent neoplasia; undiagnosed genital bleeding or a history of or active thromboembolic disorder.
   2. ERT should be initiated at the onset of menopause. Conjugated estrogens, at a dose of 0.625 mg per day, result in increases in bone density of 5%.
   3. **Bone density assessment** at regular intervals (possibly every 3-5 years) provides density data to help determine if continuation of ERT may be further recommended. If ERT is discontinued and no other therapies are instituted, serial bone density measurements should be continued to monitor bone loss.
   4. ERT doubles the risk of endometrial cancer in women with an intact uterus. This increased risk can be eliminated by the addition of medroxyprogesterone (Provera), either cyclically (12-14 days/month) at a dose of 5-10 mg, or continuously at a dose of 2.5 mg daily.
   5. Other adverse effects related to ERT are breast tenderness, weight gain, headaches, and libido changes.
D. Selective estrogen receptor modulators
   1. Selective estrogen receptor modulators (SERMs) act as estrogen analogs. Tamoxifen is approved for the prevention of breast cancer in patients with a strong family history of breast cancer. Tamoxifen prevents bone loss at the spine.
   2. **Raloxifene (Evista)**
      a. **Raloxifene** is approved for the prevention of osteoporosis. When used at 60 mg per day, raloxifene demonstrates modest increases (1.5-2% in 24 months) in bone density. This increase in density is

half of that seen in those patients receiving ERT. Raloxifene has a beneficial effect on the lipid profile similar to that seen with estrogen.
   - **b.** Raloxifene lacks breast stimulation properties, and it may provide a protective effect against breast cancer, resulting in a 50-70% reduction in breast cancer risk.
   - **c.** Minor side effects include hot flashes and leg cramps. Serious side effects include an increased risk of venous thromboembolism.

E. Bisphosphonates – alendronate (Fosamax)
   1. Alendronate is an oral bisphosphonate approved for the treatment and prevention of osteoporosis. Alendronate exerts its effect on bone by inhibiting osteoclasts.
   2. The dose for prevention of osteoporosis is 5 mg per day. This dose results in significant increases in densities of 2-3.5%, similar to those observed in ERT. The dose for treatment of osteoporosis is 10 mg per day. Alendronate provides a 50% reduction in fracture risk.
   3. Patients should take the pill in the morning with 2-3 glasses of water, at least 30 minutes before any food or beverages. No other medication should be taken at the same time, particularly calcium preparations. Patients should not lie down after taking alendronate to avoid gastroesophageal reflux. Contraindicates include severe renal insufficiency and hypocalcemia.

References: See page 140.

Infertility

Infertility is defined as failure of a couple of reproductive age to conceive after 12 months or more of regular coitus without using contraception. Infertility is considered primary when it occurs in a woman who has never established a pregnancy and secondary when it occurs in a woman who has a history of one or more previous pregnancies. Fecundability is defined as the probability of achieving a pregnancy within one menstrual cycle. It is estimated that 10% to 20% of couples are infertile.

I. Diagnostic evaluation
   A. History
      1. The history should include the couple's ages, the duration of infertility, previous infertility in other relationships, frequency of coitus, and use of lubricants (which can be spermicidal). Mumps orchitis, renal disease, radiation therapy, sexually transmitted diseases, chronic disease such as tuberculosis, major stress and fatigue, or a recent history of acute viral or febrile illness should be sought. Exposure to radiation, chemicals, excessive heat from saunas or hot tubs should be investigated.
      2. Pelvic inflammatory disease, previous pregnancies, douching practices, work exposures, alcohol and drug use, exercise, and history of any eating disorders should be evaluated.
      3. Menstrual cycle length and regularity and indirect indicators of ovulation, such as Mittelschmerz, mid-cycle cervical mucus change and premenstrual molimina, should be assessed.
   B. Physical examination for the woman
      1. Vital signs, height, and weight should be noted. Hypertension hair distribution, acne, hirsutism, thyromegaly, enlarged lymph nodes, abdominal masses or scars, galactorrhea, or acanthosis nigricans (suggestive of diabetes) should be sought.
      2. Pelvic examination should include a Papanicolaou smear and bimanual examination to assess uterine size and any ovarian masses.
      3. Testing for Chlamydia trachomatis, Mycoplasma hominis, and Ureaplasma urealyticum are recommended.

C. **Physical examination for the man**
   1. Height, weight, and hair distribution, gynecomastia, palpable lymph nodes or thyromegaly should be sought.
   2. The consistency, size, and position of both testicles and the presence of varicocele or abnormal location of the urethral meatus on the penis should be noted. Testing for Chlamydia, Ureaplasma, and Mycoplasma should be completed.
D. The cornerstone of any infertility evaluation relies on the assessment of six basic elements: (1) semen analysis, (2) sperm-cervical mucus interaction, (3) ovulation, (4) tubal patency, and (5) uterine and (6) peritoneal abnormalities. Couples of reproductive age who have intercourse regularly without contraception have approximately a 25-30% chance of conceiving in a given menstrual cycle and an 85% chance of conceiving within 1 year.
E. **Semen analysis.** The specimen is routinely obtained by masturbation and collected in a clean glass or plastic container. It is customary to have the man abstain from ejaculation for at least 2 days before producing the specimen. Criteria for a normal semen analysis include a sperm count greater than 20 million sperm/mL with at least 50% motility and 30% normal morphology.

Semen Analysis Interpretation		
Semen Parameter	Normal Values	Poor Prognosis
Sperm concentration	>20 x 10^6/mL	<5 million/ mL
Sperm motility	>50% progressive motility	<10% motility
Sperm morphology	>50% normal	<4% normal
Ejaculate volume	>2 cc	<2 cc

F. **The postcoital test (PCT)** is used to assess sperm-cervical mucus interaction after intercourse. The PCT provides information regarding cervical mucus quality and survivability of sperm after intercourse. The PCT should be performed 8 hours after intercourse and 1 to 2 days before the predicted time of ovulation, when there is maximum estrogen secretion unopposed by progesterone.
G. **Ovulation assessment**
   1. Commonly used methods used to assess ovulation include measuring a rise in basal body temperature (BBT), identifying an elevation in the midluteal phase serum progesterone concentration, luteal phase endometrial biopsy, and detection of luteinizing hormone (LH) in the urine. The BBT chart is used to acquire information regarding ovulation and the duration of the luteal phase. Female patients are instructed to take their temperature upon awaking each morning before any physical activity. A temperature rise of 0.4°F (0.22°C) for 2 consecutive days is indicative of ovulation. The initial rise in serum progesterone level occurs between 48 hours before ovulation and 24 hours after ovulation. For this reason, a rise in temperature is useful in establishing that ovulation has occurred, but it should not be used to predict the onset of ovulation in a given cycle.
   2. Another test used to assess ovulation is a midluteal phase serum progesterone concentration. A blood sample is usually obtained for progesterone 7 days after the estimated day of ovulation. A concentration greater than 3.0 ng/mL is consistent with ovulation, while a concentration greater than 10 ng/mL signifies adequate luteal phase support.
   3. Alternatively, urine LH kits can be used to assess ovulation. Unlike the

rise in BBT and serum progesterone concentrations, which are useful for retrospectively documenting ovulation, urinary LH kits can be used to predict ovulation. Ovulation usually occurs 24 to 36 hours after detecting the LH surge.
   H. **Tubal patency** can be evaluated by hysterosalpingography (HSG) and/or by chromopertubation during laparoscopy.

Timing of the Infertility Evaluation	
Test	**Day**
Hysterosalpingogram	day 7-10
Postcoital Test	day 12-14
Serum Progesterone	day 21-23
Endometrial Biopsy	day 25-28

II. Differential diagnosis and treatment
   A. The differential diagnosis of infertility includes ovarian (20%), pelvic (25%), cervical (10%), and male (35%) factors. In approximately 10% of cases no explanation is found. Optimal frequency of coitus is every other day around the time of ovulation; however, comparable pregnancy rates are achieved by 3-4 times weekly intercourse throughout the cycle.
   B. **Ovarian factor infertility**
      1. An ovarian factor is suggested by irregular cycles, abnormal BBT charts, midluteal phase serum progesterone levels less than 3 ng/mL, or luteal phase defect documented by endometrial biopsy. Ovulatory dysfunction may be intrinsic to the ovaries or caused by thyroid, adrenal, prolactin, or central nervous system disorders. Emotional stress, changes in weight, or excessive exercise should be sought because these disorders can result in ovulatory dysfunction. Luteal phase deficiency is most often the result of inadequate ovarian progesterone secretion.
      2. **Clomiphene citrate (Clomid, CC)** is the most cost-effective treatment for the treatment of infertility related to anovulation or oligo ovulation, . The usual starting dose of CC is 50 mg/day for 5 days, beginning on the second to sixth day after induced or spontaneous bleeding. Ovulation is expected between 7 and 10 days after the last dose of CC.
      3. Ovulation on a specified dosage of CC should be confirmed with a midluteal phase serum progesterone assay, BBT rise, pelvic ultrasonography, or urinary ovulation-predictor kits. In the event ovulation does not occur with a specified dose of CC, the dose can be increased by 50 mg/day in a subsequent cycle. The maximum dose of CC should not exceed 250 mg/day. The addition of dexamethasone is advocated for women with elevated dehydroepiandrosterone sulfate levels who remain anovulatory despite high doses of CC. The incidence of multiple gestations with CC is 5% to 10%. Approximately 33% of patients will become pregnant within five cycles of treatment. Treatment with CC for more than six ovulatory cycles is not recommended because of low success rates.
      4. **Human menopausal gonadotropins (hMG, Pergonal, Metrodin)** ovulation induction with is another option for the treatment of ovulatory dysfunction. Because of its expense and associated risk of multiple gestations, gonadotropin therapy should be reserved for patients who remain refractory to CC therapy. The pregnancy rate with gonadotropin therapy is 25% per cycle. This is most likely the result of recruitment of more follicles with gonadotropin therapy. The incidence of multiple

gestations with gonadotropin therapy is 25% to 30%.

5. **Luteal phase deficiency** is treated with progesterone, usually prescribed as an intravaginal suppository at a dose of 25 mg twice a day until 8 to 10 weeks of gestation.

6. **Women with ovulatory dysfunction** secondary to ovarian failure or poor ovarian reserve should consider obtaining oocytes from a donor source.

C. Pelvic factor infertility

1. Pelvic factor infertility is caused by conditions that affect the fallopian tubes, peritoneum, or uterus. Tubal factor infertility is a common sequela of salpingitis. Appendicitis, ectopic pregnancy, endometriosis, and previous pelvic or abdominal surgery can also damage the fallopian tubes and cause adhesion formation.

2. Endometriosis is another condition involving the peritoneal cavity that is commonly associated with infertility. Uterine abnormalities are responsible for infertility in about 2% of cases. Examples of uterine abnormalities associated with infertility are congenital deformities of the uterus, leiomyomas, and intrauterine scarification or adhesions (Asherman's syndrome).

3. The mainstay of treatment of pelvic factor infertility relies on laparoscopy and hysteroscopy. In many instances, tubal reconstructive surgery, lysis of adhesions, and ablation and resection of endometriosis can be accomplished laparoscopically.

D. Cervical factor infertility

1. Cervical factor infertility is suggested when well-timed PCTs are consistently abnormal in the presence of a normal semen analysis. Cervical factor infertility results from inadequate mucus production by the cervical epithelium, poor mucus quality, or the presence of antisperm antibodies.

2. Patients with an abnormal PCT should be screened for an infectious etiology. The presence of immotile sperm or sperm shaking in place and not demonstrating forward motion is suggestive of immunologically related infertility. Sperm-cervical mucus and antisperm antibody testing are indicated when PCTs are repeatedly abnormal, despite normal-appearing cervical mucus and normal semen analysis.

E. Male factor infertility includes conditions that affect sperm production, sperm maturation, and sperm delivery. Intrauterine insemination is frequently used to treat men with impaired semen parameters.

F. Unexplained Infertility

1. The term unexplained infertility should be used only after a thorough infertility investigation has failed to reveal an identifiable source and the duration of infertility is 24 months or more. History, physical examination, documentation of ovulation, endometrial biopsy, semen analyses, PCT, hysterosalpingogram, and laparoscopy should have been completed.

2. Because couples with unexplained infertility lack an identifiable causative factor of their infertility, empirical treatment with clomiphene therapy increases the spontaneous pregnancy rate to 6.8% per cycle compared with 2.8% in placebo-control cycles. For optimal results, gonadotropins should be used for ovulation induction. Intrauterine insemination, in vitro fertilization and gamete intrafallopian transfer (GIFT) are additional options.

References: See page 140.

Sexual Dysfunction

Almost two-thirds of the women may have had sexual difficulties at some time. Fifteen percent of women experience pain with intercourse, 18-48% experience difficulty becoming aroused, 46% note difficulty reaching orgasm, and 15-24% are not orgasmic.

I. **Clinical evaluation of sexual dysfunction.** Sexual difficulty can be caused by a lack of communication, insufficient stimulation, a lack of understanding of sexual response, lack of nurturing, physical discomfort, or fear of infection.

II. **Treatment of sexual dysfunction**

A. **Lack of arousal**

1. Difficulty becoming sexually aroused may occur if there is insufficient foreplay or if either partner is emotionally distracted. Arousal phase dysfunction may be manifest by insufficient vasocongestion.

2. Treatment consists of Sensate Focus exercises. In these exercises, the woman and her partner take turns caressing each other's body, except for the genital area. When caressing becomes pleasurable for both partners, they move on to manual genital stimulation, and then to further sexual activity.

B. **Lack of orgasm**

1. Lack of orgasm should be considered a problem if the patient or her partner perceives it as one. Ninety percent of women are able to experience orgasm.

2. **At-home methods of overcoming dysfunction**

a. The patient should increase self-awareness by examining her body and genitals at home. The patient should identify sensitive areas that produce pleasurable feelings. The intensity and duration of psychologic stimulation may be increased by sexual fantasy.

b. If, after completing the above steps, an orgasm has not been reached, the patient may find that the use of a vibrator on or around the clitoris is effective.

c. Once masturbation has resulted in orgasm, the patient should masturbate with her partner present and demonstrate pleasurable stimulation techniques.

d. Once high levels of arousal have been achieved, the couple may engage in intercourse. Manual stimulation of the clitoris during intercourse may be beneficial.

C. **Dyspareunia**

1. Dyspareunia consists of pain during intercourse. Organic disorders that may contribute to dyspareunia include hypoestrogenism, endometriosis, ovaries located in the cul-de-sac, fibroids, and pelvic infection.

2. Evaluation for dyspareunia should include careful assessment of the genital tract and an attempt to reproduce symptoms during bimanual examination.

D. **Vaginismus**

1. Vaginismus consists of spasm of the levator ani muscle, making penetration into the vagina painful. Some women may be unable to undergo pelvic examination.

2. **Treatment of vaginismus**

a. **Vaginal dilators.** Plastic syringe covers or vaginal dilators are available in sets of 4 graduated sizes. The smallest dilator (the size of the fifth finger) is placed in the vagina by the woman. As each dilator is replaced with the next larger size without pain, muscle relaxation occurs.

b. **Muscle awareness exercises**

(1) The examiner places one finger inside the vaginal introitus, and the woman is instructed to contract the muscle that she uses to stop urine flow. The woman then inserts her own finger into the vagina and contracts. The process is continued at home.

(2) Once a woman can identify the appropriate muscles, vaginal contractions can be done without placing a finger in the vagina.

E. Medications that interfere with sexual function. The most common of medications that interfere with sexual function are antihypertensive agents, anti-psychotics, and antidepressants.

Medications Associated With Sexual Dysfunction in Women		
Medication	**Decreased Libido**	**Delayed or No Orgasm**
Amphetamines and anorexic drugs		X
Cimetidine	X	
Diazepam		X
Fluoxetine		X
Imipramine		X
Propranolol	X	

References: See page 140.

Urinary Incontinence

Urinary incontinence is defined as the involuntary loss of urine in amounts or with sufficient frequency to constitute a social and/or health problem. The prevalence of urinary incontinence is 15 to 35 percent in community-dwelling individuals older than age 60.

I. Clinical evaluation

Urinary Incontinence: Types, Signs and Symptoms, and Causes		
Type	**Signs and symptoms**	**Causes**
Urge incontinence		
Detrusor instability (DI)	With or without urgency, usually large volume loss	Involuntary detrusor contraction, isolated or with cystitis, ureteritis, stones, neoplasia
Detrusor hyperreflexia (DI with neurologic cause)	As above, and may have urinary retention and/or vesicoureteral reflux	Central nervous system disorders: stroke, suprasacral or cord injury, parkinsonism, multiple sclerosis

Type	Signs and symptoms	Causes
Detrusor hyperreflexia with impaired contractility	Urge incontinence with elevated postvoid residual volume; must strain to empty bladder; may have symptoms of stress or overflow incontinence; episodic leakage, but frequent, moderate to large volume loss	Central nervous system disorders as above; involuntary detrusor contractions, but need to strain to empty bladder because of impaired contractility
Stress incontinence		
Stress incontinence	Small volume of urine loss with increased abdominal pressure (coughing, laughing, exercise); dry during night	Urethral hypermobility, laxity of pelvic floor muscles (common in women); weakness of urethral sphincter or bladder outlet
Intrinsic urethral sphincter deficiency	Often leak continuously or with minimal exertion	Intrinsic urethral sphincter deficiency: congenital, myelomeningocele, multiple sclerosis In women: history of surgery for urinary incontinence, estrogen deficiency, aging
Mixed incontinence (urge and stress)	Combination of urge and stress symptoms	As above; common in women
Overflow incontinence	Frequent or constant dribbling, with urge or stress symptoms	Underactive or acontractile detrusor, bladder outlet or urethral obstruction, overdistention, and overflow In women: obstruction is rare; in men: obstruction is common, eg, benign prostatic hypertrophy, neoplasm
Functional incontinence	Functional limitations interfere with ability to use the toilet	Caused by decreased physical or cognitive ability, environmental factors

History and Physical Examination in Patients with Urinary Incontinence

Urinary history
Duration of symptoms, frequency, urgency, severity
Amount of urine loss, dribbling, nocturia, hematuria, dysuria, hesitancy, weak stream, straining to void; precipitating factors (coughing, sneezing, exercise, surgery, injury)
Perineal pain, suprapubic pressure, suprapubic pain
Number of continent voids, incontinence episodes
Any previous treatment for incontinence, outcome
Use of protective devices (eg, pads, briefs)
Bladder record (voiding diary for several days)

Medical history
History of surgery, injury, pelvic radiation therapy, trauma
History of major medical illness, diabetes mellitus, congestive heart failure, peripheral edema, neurologic disease
Medications
Change in bowel habits, constipation, fecal impaction
Fluid intake, diuretic fluids (caffeine or alcohol)

Social history
Functional ability (activities of daily living, instrumental activities of daily living)
Living environment, access to toilet
Cognitive deficits, motivation

Physical examination
Orthostatic hypotension
Presence of edema that may explain nocturia or nocturnal incontinence
Neurologic diseases (eg, stroke, multiple sclerosis, spinal cord lesions; functional ability, mobility, manual dexterity; cognitive status, depression)
Abdominal examination to rule out mass, ascites, or organomegaly that might increase intra-abdominal pressure
Rectal examination to rule out mass, impaction, decreased sphincter tone, impaired sensation
Pelvic examination to evaluate for cystocele, rectocele, uterine prolapse, genital atrophy; examination for urethral diverticulum, inflammation on or carcinoma

Medications that May Contribute to Urinary Incontinence

Medications	Effect
Anticholinergics Antipsychotics Antidepressants Calcium channel blockers Antihistamines Sedative-hypnotics beta-adrenergic agonists	Urinary retention (bladder relaxation)
alpha-adrenergic agonists	Urinary retention (sphincter contraction; stress urinary incontinence symptoms improve in women)
alpha-adrenergic antagonists	Urethral relaxation (urinary incontinence symptoms improve in men with benign prostatic hypertrophy)
Diuretics Alcohol Caffeine	Polyuria

A. **Cough stress test** is performed when the woman's bladder is full, but before she has the urge to void. If there is an instantaneous, involuntary loss of urine with increased intra-abdominal pressure (cough, laugh, sneezing, exercise, Valsalva's maneuver), then stress urinary incontinence (SUI) is likely. If the loss of urine occurs after a delay or continues after the cough, then detrusor instability (DI) is suspected.

B. **Postvoid residual volume.** Portable ultrasound or catheterization can accurately measure postvoid residual (PVR) volume. PVR volume is measured a few minutes after voiding. A PVR volume less than 100 mL indicates adequate bladder emptying. A PVR volume of 100 mL or more is considered to be inadequate.

C. **Urinalysis** is performed to detect hematuria, proteinuria, glucosuria, pyuria, and bacteriuria.

D. **Other testing.** Further evaluation may include urodynamic, endoscopic, and imaging tests.

II. Etiology

A. Causes of transient incontinence include delirium; restricted mobility; retention; infection, inflammation, impaction (fecal); polyuria, pharmaceuticals).

B. Patients who have a positive cough test and consistent symptoms probably have SUI. This is the second most common type of urinary incontinence in women. A history of sudden urination of large amounts of urine suggests DI (the most common type of urinary incontinence in women), or urge incontinence. A PVR volume of more than 100 mL suggests a neurogenic bladder, especially in patients with diabetes or neurologic disease.

III. Treatment

A. Routine, or scheduled, voiding requires urinating at regular intervals (two to four hours) on a fixed schedule. In bladder training, the patient schedules voiding. This method can be very effective for stress, urge (DI) and mixed urinary incontinence.

B. Pelvic muscle exercises (PMEs), eg, Kegel exercises, are recommended for women with SUI. They may also help urge urinary incontinence. PMEs may be performed alone or with biofeedback, vaginal weights, and electrical stimulation of the pelvic floor. The patient is trained to gradually increase the duration of sustained pelvic muscle contractions to at least 10 seconds. Gradually, the number of repetitions is increased to 30 to 50 times per day for at least eight weeks.

Treatment of Urinary Incontinence

Urge incontinence
First line: behavioral and biofeedback techniques
    Bladder training
    Pelvic floor muscle exercises
    Pelvic floor electrical stimulation
    Vaginal weights
    Anticholinergic agents
    Agent of choice: Oxybutynin (Ditropan), 2.5 to 5.0 mg orally three to four times per day, or tolterodine (Detrol), 1 to 2 mg orally two times per day
    Second choice: Propantheline (Pro-Banthine), 7.5 to 30.0 mg orally three to five times per day
    Alternate: dicyclomine (eg, Bemote, Benty, Byclomine), 10 to 20 mg orally three times per day
    Imipramine (Tofranil), 10 to 25 mg orally three times per day
Second line: Surgical procedures (rarely used, recommended for intractable cases)
    Augmentation intestinocystoplasty or urinary diversion
    Bladder denervation

Stress incontinence
First line: behavioral and biofeedback techniques
Pelvic floor muscle exercises
Bladder training
Phenylpropanolamine (Entex sustained release), 25 to 100 mg orally two times per day
Pseudoephedrine (Afrin), 15 to 30 mg orally two times per day
Estrogen (oral [Premarin] or vaginal [eg, Estrace, Ogen, Premarin]), 0.3 to 1.25 mg orally once per day; 2.0 g vaginally once per day
Progestin (Provera), 2.5 to 10.0 mg orally once per day continuously or intermittently, used with estrogen in women with an intact uterus
Imipramine (Tofranil) may be use when above agents have proven unsatisfactory; 10 to 25 mg orally two times per day
Second line: surgical procedures (sometimes first line of treatment for selected women)
Procedures for hypermobility
Retropubic suspension
Needle bladder neck suspension
Anterior vaginal repair
Procedures for intrinsic sphincter deficiency
Sling procedures (intrinsic urethral sphincter deficiency with coexisting hypermobility)
Periurethral bucking injections (intrinsic urethral sphincter deficiency without hypermobility)
Placement of artificial sphincter (for intrinsic urethral sphincter deficiency with an inability to perform intermittent catheterization)

Overflow incontinence
Surgical removal of obstruction
Medication adjustments for underactive or a contractile bladder because of medication taken for other medical conditions
Intermittent catheterization for underactive detrusor muscle with or without obstruction
Indwelling catheter for women who are not candidates for surgery and those who have urinary incontinence because of urethral obstruction

C. **Pharmacologic and surgical therapies**
  1. **Urge incontinence**
     a. **Oxybutynin (Ditropan)** produces a 15-58% percent reduction in episodes of urge incontinence. It is an anticholinergic smooth-muscle relaxant. Bothersome side effects are xerostomia, blurred vision, changes in mental status, nausea, constipation, and urinary retention.
     b. **Tolterodine (Detrol)** produces a 12-18% reduction in episodes of urinary incontinence and has fewer side effects than oxybutynin.
     c. **Propantheline (Pro-Banthine)** is a second-line anticholinergic agent that produces a 13-17% reduction in incontinent episodes. High dosages are required.
  2. **Stress urinary incontinence**
     a. SUI due to sphincter insufficiency is treated with alpha-adrenergic agonists. Phenylpropanolamine or pseudoephedrine is the first line of pharmacologic therapy for women with SUI. Side effects include anxiety, insomnia, agitation, respiratory difficulty, headache, sweating, hypertension, and cardiac arrhythmia. Use caution with arrhythmias, angina, hypertension, or hyperthyroidism.
     b. **Estrogen replacement** restores urethral tone, and alpha-adrenergic response of urethral muscles. Combined therapy (estrogen and alpha-adrenergic agonists) may be more effective than alpha-adrenergic agonist therapy alone.
     c. **Imipramine** may be used in patients who do not respond to the above treatment. It has alpha-adrenergic agonist and anti-cholinergic activities and is reported to benefit women with SUI. Side effects include nausea, postural hypotension, insomnia, weakness, and fatigue.
  3. **Overflow incontinence.** If overflow incontinence is caused by an

anatomic obstruction, and the patient is an acceptable surgical candidate and has an adequately functioning detrusor muscle, then surgery to relieve the obstruction is the treatment of choice. In women, anatomic obstruction can result from severe pelvic prolapse or previous surgery for incontinence. Intermittent catheterization is the treatment of choice in patients with detrusor muscle underactivity, with or without obstruction.

References: See page 140.

Urinary Tract Infection

An estimated 40 percent of women report having had a urinary tract infections (UTI) at some point in their lives. UTIs are the leading cause of gram-negative bacteremia.

I. **Acute uncomplicated cystitis in young women**
   A. Sexually active young women have the highest risk for UTIs. Their propensity to develop UTIs is caused by a short urethra, delays in micturition, sexual activity, and the use of diaphragms and spermicides.
   B. **Symptoms of cystitis** include dysuria, urgency, and frequency without fever or back pain. Lower tract infections are most common in women in their childbearing years. Fever is absent.
   C. **A microscopic bacterial count** of 100 CFU/mL of urine has a high positive predictive value for cystitis in symptomatic women. Ninety percent of uncomplicated cystitis episodes are caused by *Escherichia coli;* 10 to 20 percent are caused by coagulase-negative *Staphylococcus saprophyticus* and 5 percent are caused by other Enterobacteriaceae organisms or enterococci. Up to one-third of uropathogens are resistant to ampicillin, but the majority are susceptible to trimethoprim-sulfamethoxazole (85 to 95 percent) and fluoroquinolones (95 percent).
   D. Young women with acute uncomplicated cystitis should receive urinalysis (examination of spun urine) and a dipstick test for leukocyte esterase.
   E. A positive leukocyte esterase test has a sensitivity of 75 to 90 percent in detecting pyuria associated with a UTI. The dipstick test for nitrite indicates bacteriuria. Enterococci, *S. saprophyticus* and Acinetobacter species produce false-negative results on nitrite testing.
   F. Three-day antibiotic regimens offer the optimal combination of convenience, low cost and efficacy comparable to seven-day or longer regimens.
   G. **Trimethoprim-sulfamethoxazole (Bactrim, Septra)**, 1 DS tab bid for 3 days, remains the antibiotic of choice in the treatment of uncomplicated UTIs in young women.
   H. A fluoroquinolone is recommended for patients who cannot tolerate sulfonamides or trimethoprim, who have a high frequency of antibiotic resistance because of recent antibiotic treatment, or who reside in an area with significant resistance to trimethoprim-sulfamethoxazole. Treatment should consist of a three-day regimen of one of the following:
      1. **Ciprofloxacin (Cipro)**, 250 mg bid.
      2. **Ofloxacin (Floxin)**, 200 mg bid.
   I. A seven-day course should be considered in pregnant women, diabetic women and women who have had symptoms for more than one week and thus are at higher risk for pyelonephritis.

II. **Recurrent cystitis in young women**
   A. Up to 20 percent of young women with acute cystitis develop recurrent UTIs. The causative organism should be identified by urine culture. Multiple infections caused by the same organism require longer courses of antibiotics and possibly further diagnostic tests. Women who have more than three UTI recurrences within one year can be managed using one of three preventive strategies:

    1. **Acute self-treatment** with a three-day course of standard therapy.
    2. **Postcoital prophylaxis** with one-half of a trimethoprim-sulfamethox-azole double-strength tablet (40/200 mg) if the UTIs have been clearly related to intercourse.
    3. **Continuous daily prophylaxis for six months:** Trimeth-oprim-sulfamethoxazole, one-half tablet/day (40/200 mg); norfloxacin (Noroxin), 200 mg/day; cephalexin (Keflex), 250 mg/day.

III. **Pyelonephritis**
  A. Acute uncomplicated pyelonephritis presents with a mild cystitis-like illness and accompanying flank pain; fever, chills, nausea, vomiting, leukocytosis and abdominal pain; or a serious gram-negative bacteremia. The microbiologic features of acute uncomplicated pyelonephritis are the same as cystitis, except that *S. saprophyticus* is a rare cause.
  B. The diagnosis should be confirmed by urinalysis with examination for pyuria and/or white blood cell casts and by urine culture. Urine cultures demonstrate more than 100,000 CFU/mL of urine. Blood cultures are positive in 20%.
  C. Oral therapy should be considered in women with mild to moderate symptoms. Since *E. coli* resistance to ampicillin, amoxicillin and first-generation cephalosporins exceeds 30 percent, these agents should not be used for the treatment of pyelonephritis. Resistance to trimethoprim-sulfamethoxazole exceeds 15 percent; therefore, empiric therapy with ciprofloxacin (Cipro), 250 mg twice daily is recommended.
  D. Patients who are too ill to take oral antibiotics should initially be treated parenterally with a third-generation cephalosporin, a broad-spectrum penicillin, a quinolone or an aminoglycoside. Once these patients have improved clinically, they can be switched to oral therapy.
  E. The total duration of therapy is usually 14 days. Patients with persistent symptoms after three days of appropriate antimicrobial therapy should be evaluated by renal ultrasonography or computed tomography for evidence of urinary obstruction. In the small percentage of patients who relapse after a two-week course, a repeated six-week course is usually curative.

IV. **Urinary tract infection in men**
  A. Urinary tract infections most commonly occur in older men with prostatic disease, outlet obstruction or urinary tract instrumentation. In men, a urine culture growing more than 1,000 CFU of a pathogen/mL of urine is the best sign of a urinary tract infection, with a sensitivity and specificity of 97 percent. Men with urinary tract infections should receive seven days of antibiotic therapy (trimethoprim-sulfamethoxazole or a fluoroquinolone).
  B. Urologic evaluation should be performed routinely in adolescents and men with pyelonephritis or recurrent infections. When bacterial prostatitis is the source of a urinary tract infection, eradication usually requires antibiotic therapy for six to 12 weeks.

References: See page 140.

Pubic Infections

I. **Human Papilloma Virus**
  A. Infections caused by human papillomavirus (HPV) account for 5.5 million, or more than one-third, of sexually transmitted diseases. More than 100 types of HPV have been identified in humans. HPV infections can cause genital warts and various benign or malignant neoplasias, or they can be entirely asymptomatic.
  B. Genital warts occur on the external genitalia and perianal area and can be visible in the vagina, on the cervix, and inside the urethra and anus. External genital warts (EGWs) are usually caused by HPV type 6 and, less commonly, by HPV type 11, both of which are considered "low-risk types" in that they are unlikely to cause squamous intraepithelial lesions (SIL) or malignancy. Approximately 15% of men and women 15-49 years of age have genital warts that can shed HPV DNA.

C. EGWs are generally visible with the naked eye and occur both in the area of the genitals and surrounding areas (ie, vulva, penis, scrotum, perianal area, perineum, pubic area, upper thighs, and crural folds). Four types of lesions occur.

1. Condyloma acuminata that are cauliflower shape and usually occur on moist surfaces.
2. Papular warts that are dome-shaped, flesh-colored, less than 4 mm in size, and occur on keratinized hair-bearing or non-hair-bearing skin.
3. Keratotic warts that have a thick, horny layer, can appear similar to common, non-genital warts, and occur on fully keratinized skin.
4. Flat-topped papules that are macular or slightly raised and occur on both moist partially keratinized or fully keratinized skin.

D. **Diagnostic approaches**
1. External warts can be diagnosed clinically with the assistance of bright light and a handheld magnifying glass. In most patients, warts have a typical appearance and are not easily confused with other skin lesions. Biopsy should be used when lesions are indurated, fixed to underlying tissue, or heavily ulcerated. Biopsy should also be considered when individual warts are greater than 1 to 2 cm, are pigmented, or respond poorly to treatment.

Treatment of External Genital Warts		
Modality	**Advantages**	**Disadvantages**
Imiquimod	Patient-applied immune response modifier	Results dependent on patient compliance; safety in pregnancy unproved
Podofilox	Patient-applied	Results dependent on patient compliance; contraindicated > 10 cm² wart area; contraindicated in pregnancy
Cryotherapy	Effective for moist and dry warts	Pain; risk of under- or over-application
Podophyllin	Most effective on moist warts	May contain mutagens; limited value for dry warts; contraindicated in pregnancy; contraindicated for large wart area; may require many applications due to low efficacy
Trichloroacetic acid/Bichloroacetic acid	Inexpensive; most effective for moist warts; safe during pregnancy	Limited value for dry warts; contraindicated for large area of friable warts; can cause burns
Curettage, electrosurgery, scissor excision	Prompt wart removal, usually in one or a few visits	Office visits; local anesthetic is usually necessary; pain is common

2. The workup for a patient presenting with EGWs should include a medical and sexual history and tests for common STDs, such as chlamydia, trichomoniasis, and bacterial vaginosis. Conditions that favor the development of EGWs include diabetes, pregnancy, and immunosuppressed states, including HIV/AIDS, lymphoproliferative disorders, and cancer chemotherapy.

E. **Treatment of external genital warts**
1. Imiquimod is the first-line patient-applied therapy because of its better clearance and lower recurrence rates compared with podofilox gel. Cryotherapy was selected as one of the first-line provider-administered therapies because of its effectiveness on both dry and moist warts found in the genital area. TCA was included as the alternate first-line provider-administered therapy in view of its effectiveness in treating warts on moist skin.
2. **Cryosurgery with liquid nitrogen or cryoprobe** is more effective than topical therapies. Lesions should be frozen until a 2 mm margin of freeze appears, then allowed to thaw, then refrozen. Repeat freeze several times.

II. **Molluscum Contagiosum**
A. This disease is produced by a virus of the pox virus family and is spread by sexual or close personal contact. Lesions are usually asymptomatic and multiple, with a central umbilication. Lesions can be spread by autoinoculation and last from 6 months to many years.
B. **Diagnosis.** The characteristic appearance is adequate for diagnosis, but biopsy may be used to confirm the diagnosis.
C. **Treatment.** Lesions are removed by sharp dermal curette, liquid nitrogen cryosurgery, or electrodesiccation.

III. **Pediculosis Pubis (Crabs)**
A. Phthirus pubis is a blood sucking louse that is unable to survive more than 24 hours off the body. It is often transmitted sexually and is principally found on the pubic hairs. Diagnosis is confirmed by locating nits or adult lice on the hair shafts.
B. **Treatment**
1. **Permethrin cream (Elimite),** 5% is the most effective treatment; it is applied for 10 minutes and washed off.
2. **Kwell shampoo,** lathered for at least 4 minutes, can also be used, but it is contraindicated in pregnancy or lactation.
3. All contaminated clothing and linen should be laundered.

IV. **Pubic Scabies**
A. This highly contagious infestation is caused by the Sarcoptes scabiei (0.2-0.4 mm in length). The infestation is transmitted by intimate contact or by contact with infested clothing. The female mite burrows into the skin, and after 1 month, severe pruritus develops. A multiform eruption may develop, characterized by papules, vesicles, pustules, urticarial wheals, and secondary infections on the hands, wrists, elbows, belt line, buttocks, genitalia, and outer feet.
B. **Diagnosis** is confirmed by visualization of burrows and observation of parasites, eggs, larvae, or red fecal compactions under microscopy.
C. **Treatment.** Permethrin 5% cream (Elimite) is massaged in from the neck down and remove by washing after 8 hours.

References: See page 140.

Sexually Transmissible Infections

Approximately 12 million patients are diagnosed with a sexually transmissible infection (STI) annually in the United States. Sequela of STIs include infertility, chronic pelvic pain, ectopic pregnancy, and other adverse pregnancy outcomes.

Diagnosis and Treatment of Bacterial Sexually Transmissible Infections

Organism	Diagnostic Methods	Recommended Treatment	Alternative
Chlamydia trachomatis	Direct fluorescent antibody, enzyme immunoassay, DNA probe, cell culture, DNA amplification	Doxycycline 100 mg PO 2 times a day for 7 days or Azithromycin (Zithromax) 1 g PO	Ofloxacin (Floxin) 300 mg PO 2 times a day for 7 days or erythromycin base 500 mg PO 4 times a day for 7 days or erythromycin ethylsuccinate 800 mg PO 4 times a day for 7 days.
Neisseria gonorrhoeae	Culture DNA probe	Ceftriaxone (Rocephin) 125 mg IM or Cefixime 400 mg PO or Ciprofloxacin (Cipro) 500 mg PO or Ofloxacin (Floxin) 400 mg PO plus Doxycycline 100 mg 2 times a day for 7 days or azithromycin 1 g PO	Single IM dose of ceftizoxime 500 mg, cefotaxime 500 mg, cefotetan 1 g, and cefoxitin (Mefoxin) 2 g with probenecid 1 g PO; or enoxacin 400 mg PO, lomefloxacin 400 mg PO, or norfloxacin 800 mg PO
Treponema pallidum	Clinical appearance Dark-field microscopy Nontreponemal test: rapid plasma reagin, VDRL Treponemal test: MHA-TP, FTA-ABS	Primary and secondary syphilis and early latent syphilis (<1 year duration): benzathine penicillin G 2.4 million units IM in a single dose.	Penicillin allergy in patients with primary, secondary, or early latent syphilis (<1 year of duration): doxycycline 100 mg PO 2 times a day for 2 weeks.

Diagnosis and Treatment of Viral Sexually Transmissible Infections

Organism	Diagnostic Methods	Recommended Treatment Regimens
Herpes simplex virus	Clinical appearance Cell culture confirmation	First episode: Acyclovir (Zovirax) 400 mg PO 5 times a day for 7-10 days, or famciclovir (Famvir) 250 mg PO 3 times a day for 7-10 days, or valacyclovir (Valtrex) 1 g PO 2 times a day for 7-10 days. Recurrent episodes: acyclovir 400 mg PO 3 times a day for 5 days, or 800 mg PO 2 times a day for 5 days or famciclovir 125 mg PO 2 times a day for 5 days or valacyclovir 500 mg PO 2 times a day for 5 days Daily suppressive therapy: acyclovir 400 mg PO 2 times a day, or famciclovir 250 mg PO 2 times a day, or valacyclovir 250 mg PO 2 times a day, 500 mg PO 1 time a day, or 1000 mg PO 1 time a day

Organism	Diagnostic Methods	Recommended Treatment Regimens
Human papilloma virus	Clinical appearance of condyloma papules Cytology	External warts: Patient may apply podofilox 0.5% solution or gel 2 times a day for 3 days, followed by 4 days of no therapy, for a total of up to 4 cycles, or imiquimod 5% cream at bedtime 3 times a week for up to 16 weeks. Cryotherapy with liquid nitrogen or cryoprobe, repeat every 1-2 weeks; or podophyllin, repeat weekly; or TCA 80-90%, repeat weekly; or surgical removal. Vaginal warts: cryotherapy with liquid nitrogen, or TCA 80-90%, or podophyllin 10-25%
Human immuno-deficiency virus	Enzyme immunoassay Western blot (for confirmation) Polymerase chain reaction	Antiretroviral agents

Treatment of Pelvic Inflammatory Disease		
Regimen	Inpatient	Outpatient
A	Cefotetan (Cefotan) 2 g IV q12h; or cefoxitin (Mefoxin) 2 g IV q6h plus doxycycline 100 mg IV or PO q12h.	Ofloxacin (Floxin) 400 mg PO bid for 14 days plus metronidazole 500 mg PO bid for 14 days.
B	Clindamycin 900 mg IV q8h plus gentamicin loading dose IV or IM (2 mg/kg of body weight), followed by a maintenance dose (1.5 mg/kg) q8h.	Ceftriaxone (Rocephin) 250 mg IM once; or cefoxitin 2 g IM plus probenecid 1 g PO; or other parenteral third-generation cephalosporin (eg, ceftizoxime, cefotaxime) plus doxycycline 100 mg PO bid for 14 days.

I. **Chlamydia trachomatis**
   A. Chlamydia trachomatis is the most prevalent STI in the United States. Chlamydial infections are most common in women age 15-19 years.
   B. Routine screening of asymptomatic, sexually active adolescent females undergoing pelvic examination is recommended. Annual screening should be done for women age 20-24 years who are either inconsistent users of barrier contraceptives or who acquired a new sex partner or had more than one sexual partner in the past 3 months.
II. **Gonorrhea.** Gonorrhea has an incidence of 800,000 cases annually. Routine screening for gonorrhea is recommended among women at high risk of infection, including prostitutes, women with a history of repeated episodes of gonorrhea, women under age 25 years with two or more sex partners in the past year, and women with mucopurulent cervicitis.
III. **Syphilis**
   A. Syphilis has an incidence of 100,000 cases annually. The rates are highest in the South, among African Americans, and among those in the 20- to 24-year-old age group.
   B. Prostitutes, persons with other STIs, and sexual contacts of persons with active syphilis should be screened.
IV. **Herpes simplex virus and human papillomavirus**
   A. An estimated 200,000-500,000 new cases of herpes simplex occur annually in the United States. New infections are most common in adolescents and young adults.

B. Human papillomavirus affects about 30% of young, sexually active individuals.
References: See page 140.

Pelvic Inflammatory Disease

Pelvic inflammatory disease (PID) represents a spectrum of infections and inflammatory disorders of the uterus, fallopian tubes, and adjacent pelvic structures. PID may include any combination of endometritis, salpingitis, tubo-ovarian abscess, oophoritis, and in its more extreme manifestation, pelvic peritonitis. One out of every 10 women will have at least one episode of PID during her reproductive years. At least one-quarter of women with PID will have major complications, including infertility, ectopic pregnancy, chronic pelvic pain, tubo-ovarian abscesses, and/or pelvic adhesions.

I. Etiology and clinical pathogenesis

A. PID results when pathogenic microorganisms spread from the cervix and vagina to the upper portions of the genital tract to such structures as the salpinx, ovaries, and adjacent structures. Chlamydia has been shown to be responsible for 25-50% of all cases of PID. About 10-20% of female patients who are infected with gonorrhea will progress to PID.

B. Mixed infections are responsible for up to 70% of cases with PID. These polymicrobial infections typically include both anaerobic and aerobic microorganisms. Anaerobes such as Bacteroides, Peptostreptococcus, and Peptococcus have been reported, as have facultative bacteria, including Gardnerella vaginalis, Streptococcus, E. coli, and Haemophilus influenzae.

C. PID occurs almost exclusively in sexually active women and is most common in adolescents. Risk factors include sexual activity, particularly with multiple sexual partners, young age, and use of an intrauterine device. Oral contraceptive users have a lower risk for developing PID.

II. Diagnosis and evaluation

A. Presumptive diagnosis of PID is made in women who are sexually active who present with lower abdominal pain and cervical, uterine, or adnexal tenderness on pelvic examination. The CDC has recommended minimum criteria required for empiric treatment of PID. These major determinants include lower abdominal tenderness, adnexal tenderness, and cervical motion tenderness. Minor determinants (ie, signs that may increase the suspicion of PID) include:

1. Fever (oral temperature >101°F; >38.3°C)
2. Vaginal discharge
3. Documented STD
4. Erythrocyte sedimentation rate (ESR)
5. C-reactive protein
6. Systemic signs
7. Dyspareunia

Laboratory Evaluation for Pelvic Inflammatory Disease

- Complete blood count with differential
- Pregnancy test
- Tests for Chlamydia and gonorrhea
- RPR or VDRL tests for syphilis

Differential Diagnosis of Pelvic Inflammatory Disease	
Appendicitis	Irritable bowel syndrome
Ectopic pregnancy	Somatization
Hemorrhagic ovarian cyst	Gastroenteritis
Ovarian torsion	Cholecystitis
Endometriosis	Nephrolithiasis
Urinary tract Infection	

III. **Management**
   A. A high index of suspicion and a low threshold for initiating treatment are important for facilitating detection and appropriate management of PID for all women of child-bearing age with pelvic pain. Laparoscopy is seldom practical. Antibiotic therapy is usually initiated on clinical grounds. Lower abdominal tenderness, adnexal tenderness, and pain on manipulation of the cervix mandates treatment.

Antibiotic Treatment of Hospitalized Patients with Pelvic Inflammatory Disease

Inpatient Parenteral Regimen One
Azithromycin (Zithromax) IV (500 mg qd for 1 or 2 days) followed by oral azithromycin 250 mg po once daily to complete a total of 7 days
Plus (as clinically indicated for suspicion for anaerobic infection)
Metronidazole (Flagyl) 500 mg IV every 8 hours

Inpatient Parenteral Regimen Option Two
Cefotetan (Cefotan) 2 g IV every 12 hours
   Plus
Doxycycline 100 mg IV or po every 12 hours
   or
Cefoxitin (Mefoxin) 2 g IV every 6 hours
   Plus
Doxycycline 100 mg IV or PO every 12 hours
Parenteral therapy can be discontinued 24 hours after the patient improves. Oral therapy should be started with doxycycline 100 mg bid and continued for 14 days total therapy. If a tubo-ovarian abscess is present, clindamycin or metronidazole should be used.

Inpatient Parenteral Regimen Option Three
Clindamycin 900 mg IV every 8 hours
   Plus
Gentamicin 2mg/kg loading dose IV or IM (with 1.5 mg/kg maintenance dose every 8 hours)
Parenteral therapy can be discontinued 24 hours after the patient improves. Oral therapy should then be continued for a total of 14 days of therapy. Oral therapy should consist of doxycycline 100 mg bid and clindamycin 450 mg qid.

Alterative Parenteral Regimen Options
Ofloxacin (Floxin) 400 mg IV every 12 hours
   Plus
Metronidazole (Flagyl) 500 mg IV every 8 hours
   or
Ampicillin/sulbactam (Unasyn) 3 g IV every 6 hours
   Plus
Doxycycline 100 mg PO or IV every 12 hours
   or
Ciprofloxacin (Cipro) 200 mg IV every 12 hours
   Plus
Doxycycline 100 mg PO or IV every 12 hours
   Plus
Metronidazole (Flagyl) 500 mg IV every 8 hours

Outpatient Treatment of Pelvic Inflammatory Disease

Azithromycin (Zithromax) 500 mg as a single dose intravenously (2 mg/mL over 1 hour) followed by oral azithromycin 250 mg once daily orally to complete a total of seven days of therapy.
Plus/Minus
Metronidazole (Flagyl) 500 mg orally twice daily for 14 days.

Ceftriaxone (Rocephin) 250 mg IM once
   Plus
Doxycycline 100 mg orally twice daily for 14 days
   Plus/Minus
Metronidazole (Flagyl) 500 mg orally twice daily for 14 days

Cefoxitin (Mefoxin) 2 g IM plus probenecid 1 gram orally concurrently
   Plus
Doxycycline 100 mg orally twice daily for 14 days
   Plus/Minus
Metronidazole (Flagyl) 500 mg orally twice daily for 14 days

Ofloxacin (Floxin) 400 mg orally twice daily for 14 days
   Plus
Metronidazole (Flagyl) 500 mg orally twice daily for 14 days

   B. Male sexual partners of patients with PID should be evaluated for sexually transmitted infections, and they must be treated for chlamydial and gonococcal disease.

References: See page 140.

Vaginitis

Vaginitis is the most common gynecologic problem encountered by primary care physicians. It may result from bacterial infections, fungal infection, protozoan infection, contact dermatitis, atrophic vaginitis, or allergic reaction.

I. Pathophysiology
   A. Vaginitis results from alterations in the vaginal ecosystem, either by the introduction of an organism or by a disturbance that allows normally present pathogens to proliferate.
   B. Antibiotics may cause the overgrowth of yeast. Douching may alter the pH level or selectively suppress the growth of endogenous bacteria.
II. Clinical evaluation of vaginal symptoms
   A. The type and extent of symptoms, such as itching, discharge, odor, or pelvic pain should be determined. A change in sexual partners or sexual activity, changes in contraception method, medications (antibiotics), and history of prior genital infections should be sought.
   B. Physical examination
      1. Evaluation of the vagina should include close inspection of the external genitalia for excoriations, ulcerations, blisters, papillary structures, erythema, edema, mucosal thinning, or mucosal pallor.
      2. The color, texture, and odor of vaginal or cervical discharge should be noted.
   C. Vaginal fluid pH can be determined by immersing pH paper in the vaginal discharge. A pH level greater than 4.5 often indicates the presence of bacterial vaginosis or Trichomonas vaginalis.
   D. Saline wet mount
      1. One swab should be used to obtain a sample from the posterior vaginal fornix, obtaining a "clump" of discharge. Place the sample on

     a slide, add one drop of normal saline, and apply a coverslip.

    2. Coccoid bacteria and clue cells (bacteria-coated, stippled, epithelial cells) are characteristic of bacterial vaginosis.

    3. Trichomoniasis is confirmed by identification of trichomonads--mobile, oval flagellates. White blood cells are prevalent.

E. **Potassium hydroxide (KOH) preparation**

    1. Place a second sample on a slide, apply one drop of 10% potassium hydroxide (KOH) and a coverslip. A pungent, fishy odor upon addition of KOH--a positive whiff test--strongly indicates bacterial vaginosis.

    2. The KOH prep may reveal Candida in the form of thread-like hyphae and budding yeast.

F. **Screening for STDs.** Testing for gonorrhea and chlamydial infection should be completed for women with a new sexual partner, purulent cervical discharge, or cervical motion tenderness.

III. **Differential diagnosis**

A. The most common cause of vaginitis is bacterial vaginosis, followed by Candida albicans. The prevalence of trichomoniasis has declined in recent years.

B. Common nonvaginal etiologies include contact dermatitis from spermicidal creams, latex in condoms, or douching. Any STD can produce vaginal discharge.

Clinical Manifestations of Vaginitis	
Candidal Vaginitis	Nonmalodorous, thick, white, "cottage cheese-like" discharge that adheres to vaginal walls Presence of hyphal forms or budding yeast cells on wet-mount Pruritus Normal pH (<4.5)
Bacterial Vaginosis	Thin, dark or dull grey, homogeneous, malodorous discharge that adheres to the vaginal walls Elevated pH level (>4.5) Positive KOH (whiff test) Clue cells on wet-mount microscopic evaluation
Trichomonas Vaginalis	Copious, yellow-gray or green, homogeneous or frothy, malodorous discharge Elevated pH level (>4.5) Mobile, flagellated organisms and leukocytes on wet-mount microscopic evaluation Vulvovaginal irritation, dysuria
Atrophic Vaginitis	Vaginal dryness or burning

IV. **Bacterial Vaginosis**

A. Bacterial vaginosis develops when a shift in the normal vaginal ecosystem causes replacement of the usually predominant lactobacilli with mixed bacterial flora. Bacterial vaginosis is the most common type of vaginitis. It is found in 10-25% of patients in gynecologic clinics.

B. There is usually little itching, no pain, and the symptoms tend to have an indolent course. A malodorous fishy vaginal discharge is characteristic.

C. There is usually little or no inflammation of the vulva or vaginal epithelium. The vaginal discharge is thin, dark or dull grey, and homogeneous.

D. A wet-mount will reveal clue cells (epithelial cells stippled with bacteria), an abundance of bacteria, and the absence of homogeneous bacilli (lactobacilli).

E. **Diagnostic criteria** (3 of 4 criterial present)

    1. pH >4.0

    2. Clue cells

    3. Positive KOH whiff test

    4. Homogeneous discharge.
- **F. Treatment regimens**
  - **1. Topical (intravaginal) regimens**
    - **a.** Metronidazole gel (MetroGel) 0.75%, one applicatorful (5 g) bid 5 days.
    - **b.** Clindamycin cream (Cleocin) 2%, one applicatorful (5 g) qhs for 7 nights. Topical therapies have a 90% cure rate.
  - **2. Oral metronidazole (Flagyl)**
    - **a.** Oral metronidazole is equally effective as topical therapy, with a 90% cure rate.
    - **b.** Dosage is 500 mg bid or 250 mg tid for 7 days. A single 2-g dose is slightly less effective (69-72%) and causes more gastrointestinal upset. Alcohol products should be avoided because nausea and vomiting (disulfiram reaction) may occur.
  - **3.** Routine treatment of sexual partners is not necessary, but it is sometimes helpful for patients with frequent recurrences.
  - **4. Persistent cases** should be reevaluated and treated with clindamycin, 300 mg PO bid for 7 days along with treatment of sexual partners.
  - **5. Pregnancy.** Clindamycin is recommended, either intravaginally as a daily application of 2% cream or PO, 300 mg bid for 7 days. After the first trimester, oral or topical therapy with metronidazole is acceptable.

V. Candida Vulvovaginitis
- **A.** Candida is the second most common diagnosis associated with vaginal symptoms. It is found in 25% of asymptomatic women. Fungal infections account for 33% of all vaginal infections.
- **B.** Patients with diabetes mellitus or immunosuppressive conditions such as infection with the HIV are at increased risk for candidal vaginitis. Candidal vaginitis occurs in 25-70% of women after antibiotic therapy.
- **C.** The most common symptom is pruritus. Vulvar burning and an increase or change in consistency of the vaginal discharge may be noted.
- **D. Physical examination**
  - **1.** Candidal vaginitis causes a nonmalodorous, thick, adherent, white vaginal discharge that appears "cottage cheese-like."
  - **2.** The vagina is usually hyperemic and edematous. Vulvar erythema may be present.
- **E.** The normal pH level is not usually altered with candidal vaginitis. Microscopic examination of vaginal discharge diluted with saline (wet-mount) and 10% KOH preparations will reveal hyphal forms or budding yeast cells. Some yeast infections are not detected by microscopy because there are relatively few numbers of organisms. Confirmation of candidal vaginitis by culture is not recommended. Candida on Pap smear is not a sensitive finding because the yeast is a constituent of the normal vaginal flora.
- **F. Treatment of candida vulvovaginitis**
  - **1.** For severe symptoms and chronic infections, a 7-day course of treatment is used, instead of a 1- or 3-day course. If vulvar involvement is present, a cream should be used instead of a suppository.
  - **2.** Most C. albicans isolates are susceptible to either clotrimazole or miconazole. An increasing number of nonalbicans Candida species are resistant to the OTC antifungal agents and require the use of prescription antifungal agents. Greater activity has been achieved using terconazole, butoconazole, tioconazole, ketoconazole, and fluconazole.

Antifungal Medications		
Medication	**How Supplied**	**Dosage**
Prescription Agents Oral Agents		
Fluconazole (Diflucan)	150-mg tablet	1 tablet PO 1 time
Ketoconazole (Nizoral)	200 mg	1 tablet PO bid for 5 days
Prescription Topical Agents		
Butoconazole (Femstat)	2% vaginal cream [28 g]	1 vaginally applicatorful qhs for 3 nights
Clotrimazole (Gyne-Lotrimin)	500-mg tablet	1 tablet vaginally qhs 1 time
Miconazole (Monistat 3)	200-mg vaginal suppositories	1 suppository vaginally qhs for 3 nights
Tioconazole (Vagistat)	6.5% cream [5 g]	1 applicatorful vaginally qhs 1 time
Terconazole (Terazol 3)	Cream: 0.4% [45 gm]	One applicatorful intravaginally qhs x 7 days
	Cream: 0.8% [20 gm]	One applicatorful intravaginally qhs x 3 days
	Vag suppository: 80 mg [3]	One suppository intravaginally qhs x 3 days
Over-the-Counter Agents		
Clotrimazole (Gyne-Lotrimin)	1% vaginal cream [45 g] 100-mg vaginal tablets	1 applicatorful vaginally qhs for 7-14 nights 1 tablet vaginally qhs for 7-14 days
Miconazole (Monistat 7)	2% cream [45 g] 100-mg vaginal suppository	1 applicatorful vaginally qhs for 7 days 1 suppository vaginally qhs for 7 days

    3. Ketoconazole, 200-mg oral tablets twice daily for 5 days, is effective in treating resistant and recurrent candidal infections. Effectiveness is results from the elimination of the rectal reservoir of yeast.

    4. Resistant infections also may respond to vaginal boric acid, 600 mg in size 0 gelatin capsules daily for 14 days.

    5. Treatment of male partners is usually not necessary but may be considered if the partner has yeast balanitis or is uncircumcised.

    6. During pregnancy, butoconazole (Femstat) should be used in the 2nd or 3rd trimester. Miconazole or clotrimazole may also be used.

G. Resistant or recurrent cases

    1. Recurrent infections should be reevaluated. Repeating topical therapy for a 14- to 21-day course may be effective. Oral regimens have the potential for eradicating rectal reservoirs.

    2. Cultures are helpful in determining whether a non-candidal species is present. Patients with recalcitrant disease should be evaluated for diabetes and HIV.

VI. Trichomonas Vaginalis
  A. Trichomonas, a flagellated anaerobic protozoan, is a sexually transmitted disease with a high transmission rate. Non-sexual transmission is possible because the organism can survive for a few hours in a moist environment.
  B. A copious, yellow-gray or green homogeneous discharge is present. A foul odor, vulvovaginal irritation, and dysuria is common. The pH level is usually greater than 4.5.
  C. The diagnosis of trichomonal infection is made by examining a wet-mount preparation for mobile, flagellated organisms and an abundance of leukocytes. Occasionally the diagnosis is reported on a Pap test, and treatment is recommended.
  D. Treatment of Trichomonas vaginalis
    1. Metronidazole (Flagyl), 2 g PO in a single dose for both the patient and sexual partner, or 500 mg PO bid for 7 days.
    2. Topical therapy with topical metronidazole is not recommended because the organism may persist in the urethra and Skene's glands. Screening for coexisting sexually transmitted diseases should be completed.
    3. **Recurrent or recalcitrant infections**
      a. If patients are compliant but develop recurrent infections, treatment of their sexual partners should be confirmed.
      b. Cultures should be performed. In patients with persistent infection, a resistant trichomonal strain may require high dosages of metronidazole of 2.5 g/d, often combined with intravaginal metronidazole for 10 days.

VII. Other diagnoses causing vaginal symptoms
  A. One-third of patients with vaginal symptoms will not have laboratory evidence of bacterial vaginosis, Candida, or Trichomonas. Other causes of the vaginal symptoms include cervicitis, allergic reactions, and vulvodynia.
  B. **Atrophic vaginitis** should be considered in postmenopausal patients if the mucosa appears pale and thin and wet-mount findings are negative.
    1. Oral estrogen (Premarin) 0.625 mg qd should provide relief.
    2. Estradiol vaginal cream 0.01% may be effective as 2-4 g daily for 1-2 weeks, then 1 g, one to three times weekly.
    3. Conjugated estrogen vaginal cream (Premarin) may be effective as 2-4 g daily (3 weeks on, 1 week off) for 3-6 months.
  C. **Allergy and chemical irritation**
    1. Patients should be questioned about use of substances that cause allergic or chemical irritation, such as deodorant soaps, laundry detergent, vaginal contraceptives, bath oils, perfumed or dyed toilet paper, hot tub or swimming pool chemicals, and synthetic clothing.
    2. Topical steroids and systemic antihistamines can help alleviate the symptoms.

References: See page 140.

Gynecologic Oncology

Cervical Cancer

About 12,800 women in the United States developed cancer of the uterine cervix each year, and about 4,800 women died of the disease. The incidence of cervical cancer has dramatically decreased from 32 cases per 100,000 women in the 1940s to 8.3 cases per 100,000 women in the 1980s. Women who are at risk for developing cellular abnormalities include those who smoke and those with a history of sexually transmitted diseases, human papillomavirus (HPV) infection, low socioeconomic status, two or more lifetime sexual partners or immunosuppression.

I. **Cytologic screening**
   A. All women should receive screening Pap smears at the onset of sexual activity or at 18 years of age, because strong evidence supports the theory that routine screening with Pap smears will lower the rate of cervical cancer.
   B. Once three normal annual Pap smears are documented, the interval for continued surveillance with screening Pap smears may be lengthened. Pap smears that suggest invasive disease require further evaluation by colposcopy, colposcopic-directed biopsy and endocervical curettage.

International Federation of Gynecologists and Obstetricians Staging System for Cervical Cancer	
Stage	**Characteristics**
0	Carcinoma in situ, intraepithelial neoplasia.
I	Carcinoma strictly confined to the cervix.
Ia	Invasive cancer identified only microscopically. All gross lesions, even with superficial invasion, are stage Ib cancers. Invasion is limited to measured invasion of stroma ≤5 mm in depth and ≤7 mm in width.
Ia1	Measured invasion of stroma ≤3 mm in depth and ≤7 mm in width.
Ia2	Measured invasion of stroma >3 mm and ≤5 mm in depth and ≤7mm in width.
Ib	Clinical lesions confined to the cervix or preclinical lesions greater than Ia.
Ib1	Clinical lesions ≤4cm in size.
Ib2	Clinical lesions >4cm in size.
II	Carcinoma extends beyond the cervix but not to the pelvic wall; carcinoma involves the vagina but not as far as the lower one third.
IIa	No obvious parametrial involvement.
IIb	Obvious parametrial involvement.

III	Carcinoma has extended to the pelvic wall; on rectal examination no cancer-free space is found between the tumor and the pelvic wall; the tumor involves the lower one third of the vagina; all cases with a hydronephrosis or nonfunctioning kidney should be included, unless they are known to be related to another cause.
IIIa	No extension to the pelvic wall, but involvement of the lower one third of the vagina.
IIIb	Extension to the pelvic wall and hydronephrosis or nonfunctioning kidney, or both.
IV	Carcinoma has extended beyond the true pelvis or has clinically involved the mucosa of the bladder or rectum.
IVa	Spread to adjacent organs.
IVb	Spread to distant organs.

II. Management

- **A.** Once the diagnosis of invasive cervical cancer is established by histology, the disease is clinically staged.
- **B.** Pretreatment evaluation includes taking a thorough history and conducting a physical examination. Particular emphasis should be placed on the pelvic examination, because cervical cancer is often locally destructive before it is metastatic. A rectovaginal examination is important to identify nodules or masses that indicate the possibility of locally invasive disease.

Pretreatment Assessment of Women with Histologic Diagnosis of Cervical Cancer

History
Physical examination
Complete blood count, blood urea nitrogen, creatinine, hepatic function
Chest radiography
Intravenous pyelography or computed tomography of abdomen with intravenous contrast
Consider the following: barium enema, cystoscopy, rectosigmoidoscopy

---

- **C.** Selective use of chest radiography, intravenous pyelography, cystoscopy, gastrointestinal endoscopy (ie, flexible sigmoidoscopy), lymphangiography, computed tomography (CT) or magnetic resonance imaging (MRI) of the pelvis and abdomen may be useful in appraising the degree of metastatic disease. Assessment of renal function is vital to the staging of cervical cancer. The presence of unilateral or bilateral ureteral obstruction with azotemia often heralds metastatic disease and heralds a poorer prognosis.
- **D. Stage Ia tumors**
  1. Stage Ia tumors are first diagnosed by colposcopic-directed biopsy and are confirmed by cone biopsy. The prognosis is good. Five-year survival exceeds 95 percent with appropriate treatment.
  2. Therapy is simple hysterectomy without pelvic lymph node dissection. Adequate cone biopsy with close follow-up is an option in women who wish to preserve their fertility and understand the potential risk of progression.
- **E. Stage Ib and IIa tumors** are diagnosed clinically and can be treated surgically or with radiotherapy. Both treatments produce similar results, with a five-year survival rate of 80 to 90 percent. Surgery includes a radical hysterectomy. Oophorectomy is not necessary in premenopausal women.
- **F. Stage IIb, III and IV tumors.** Once the tumor extends to or invades local organs, radiation therapy becomes the mainstay of treatment. This therapy provides five-year survival rates of 65, 40 and less than 20 percent for

stages IIb, III and IV, respectively. Patients with distant metastases (stage IVb) also require chemotherapy to control systemic disease.
References: See page 140.

Endometrial Cancer

Uterine cancer is the most common malignant neoplasm of the female genital tract and the fourth most common cancer in women. About 6,000 women in the United States die of this disease each year. It is more frequent in affluent and white, especially obese, postmenopausal women of low parity. Hypertension and diabetes mellitus are also predisposing factors.

I. Risk factors
A. Any characteristic that increases exposure to unopposed estrogen increases the risk for endometrial cancer. Conversely, decreasing exposure to estrogen limits the risk. Unopposed estrogen therapy, obesity, anovulatory cycles and estrogen-secreting neoplasms all increase the amount of unopposed estrogen and thereby increase the risk for endometrial cancer. Smoking seems to decrease estrogen exposure, thereby decreasing the cancer risk, and oral contraceptive use increases progestin levels, thus providing protection.
B. **Hormone replacement therapy.** Unopposed estrogen treatment of menopause is associated with an eightfold increased incidence of endometrial cancer. The addition of progestin decreases this risk dramatically.

Risk Factors for Endometrial Cancer
Unopposed estrogen exposure
Median age at diagnosis: 59 years
Menstrual cycle irregularities, specifically menorrhagia and menometrorrhagia
Postmenopausal bleeding
Chronic anovulation
Nulliparity
Early menarche (before 12 years of age)
Late menopause (after 52 years of age)
Infertility
Tamoxifen (Nolvadex) use
Granulosa and thecal cell tumors
Ovarian dysfunction
Obesity
Diabetes mellitus
Arterial hypertension with or without atherosclerotic heart disease
History of breast or colon cancer

II. Clinical evaluation
A. Ninety percent of patients with endometrial cancer have abnormal vaginal bleeding, usually presenting as menometrorrhagia in a perimenopausal woman or menstrual-like bleeding in a woman past menopause. Perimenopausal women relate a history of intermenstrual bleeding, excessive bleeding lasting longer than seven days or an interval of less than 21 days between menses. Heavy, prolonged bleeding in patients known to be at risk for anovulatory cycles should prompt histologic evaluation of the endometrium. The size, contour, mobility and position of the uterus should be noted.
B. Patients who report abnormal vaginal bleeding and have risk factors for endometrial cancer should have histologic evaluation of the endometrium. Premenopausal patients with amenorrhea for more than six to 12 months should be offered endometrial sampling, especially if they have risk factors associated with excessive estrogen exposure. Postmenopausal women with vaginal bleeding who either are not on hormonal replacement therapy

or have been on therapy longer than six months should be evaluated by endometrial sampling.

C. Endometrial sampling

1. In-office sampling of the endometrial lining may be accomplished with a Novak or Kevorkian curet, the Pipelle endometrial-suction curet, or the Vabra aspirator. Before having an in-office biopsy, the patient should take a preoperative dose of a nonsteroidal anti-inflammatory drug (NSAID). With the patient in the lithotomy position, a speculum is inserted in the vaginal canal. The cervix should be cleansed with a small amount of an antiseptic solution. After 1 mL of a local anesthetic is infused into the anterior lip of the cervix, a tenaculum is placed. The paracervical block is then performed using 1 or 2 percent lidocaine (Xylocaine) without epinephrine.

2. The cannula is then placed in the uterus and placement is confirmed with the help of the centimeter markings along the cannula. The inner sleeve is then pulled back while the cannula is held within the cavity. This generates a vacuum in the cannula that can be used to collect endometrial tissue for diagnosis. Moving the cannula in and out of the cavity no more than 2 to 3 cm with each stroke while turning the cannula clockwise or counterclockwise is helpful in obtaining specimens from the entire cavity.

III. Treatment of endometrial cancer

A. The treatment of endometrial cancer is usually surgical, such as total abdominal hysterectomy, bilateral salpingo-oophorectomy and evaluation for metastatic disease, which may include pelvic or para-aortic lymphadenectomy, peritoneal cytologic examination and peritoneal biopsies. The extent of the surgical procedure is based on the stage of disease, which can be determined only at the time of the operation.

Staging for Carcinoma of the Corpus Uteri	
Stage*	**Description**
IA (G1, G2, G3)	Tumor limited to endometrium
IB (G1, G2, G3)	Invasion of less than one half of the myometrium
IC (G1, G2, G3)	Invasion of more than one half of the myometrium
IIA (G1, G2, G3)	Endocervical gland involvement
IIB (G1, G2, G3)	Cervical stromal involvement
IIIA (G1, G2, G3)	Invasion of serosa and/or adnexa and/or positive peritoneal cytologic results
IIIB (G1, G2, G3)	Metastases to vagina
IIIC (G1, G2, G3)	Metastases to pelvic and/or para-aortic lymph nodes
IVA (G1, G2, G3)	Invasion of bladder and/or bowel mucosa

| IVB | Distant metastases including intra-abdominal and/or inguinal lymph nodes |

*--Carcinoma of the corpus is graded (G) according to the degree of histologic differentiation: G1 = 5 percent or less of a solid growth pattern; G2 = 6 to 50 percent of a solid growth pattern; G3 = more than 50 percent of a solid growth pattern.

- **B.** For most patients whose cancers have progressed beyond stage IB grade 2, postoperative radiation therapy is recommended. Because tumor response to cytotoxic chemotherapy has been poor, chemotherapy is used only for palliation.
- **C.** Endometrial hyperplasia with atypia should be treated with hysterectomy except in extraordinary cases. Progestin treatment is a possibility in women younger than 40 years of age who refuse hysterectomy or who wish to retain their childbearing potential, but an endometrial biopsy should be performed every three months. Treatment of atypical hyperplasia and well-differentiated endometrial cancer with progestins in women younger than 40 years of age results in complete regression of disease in 94 percent and 75 percent, respectively.
- **D.** Patients found to have hyperplasia without atypia should be treated with progestins and have an endometrial biopsy every three to six months.
- IV. **Serous and clear cell adenocarcinomas**
  - **A.** These cancers are considered in a separate category from endometrioid adenocarcinomas. They have a worse prognosis overall. Patients with serious carcinomas have a poorer survival. The 3 year survival is 40% for stage I disease.
  - **B.** Serous and clear cell carcinomas are staged like ovarian cancer. A total abdominal hysterectomy and bilateral salpingo-oophorectomy, lymph node biopsy, and omental biopsy/omentectomy are completed. Washings from the pelvis, gutters and diaphragm are obtained, and the diaphragm is sampled and peritoneal biopsies completed.

References: See page 140.

Ovarian Cancer

A woman has a 1-in-70 risk of developing ovarian cancer in her lifetime. The incidence is 1.4 per 100,000 women under age 40, increasing to approximately 45 per 100,000 for women over age 60. The median age at diagnosis is 61. A higher incidence of ovarian cancer is seen in women who have never been pregnant or who are of low parity. Women who have had either breast or colon cancer or have a family history of these cancers also are at higher risk of developing ovarian cancer. Protective factors include multiparity, oral contraceptive use, a history of breastfeeding, and anovulatory disorders.

- I. **Screening.** There is no proven method of screening for ovarian cancer. Routine screening by abdominal or vaginal ultrasound or measurement of CA 125 levels in serum cannot be recommended for women with no known risk factors. For women with familial ovarian cancer syndrome who wish to maintain their reproductive capacity, transvaginal ultrasonography, analysis of levels of CA 125 in serum, or both, in combination with frequent pelvic examinations may be considered.
- II. **Diagnosis**
  - **A.** **History.** There are no early symptoms of cancer of the ovary. Abdominal discomfort, upper abdominal fullness, and early satiety are associated with cancer of the ovary. Other frequently encountered signs and symptoms are fatigue, increasing abdominal girth, urinary frequency, and shortness of breath caused by pleural effusion or massive ascites.
  - **B.** **Physical findings.** The most frequently noted physical finding of ovarian

cancer is a pelvic mass. An adnexal mass that is bilateral, irregular, solid, or fixed suggests malignancy. Other findings suggestive of malignancy are ascites or a nodular cul-de-sac. The risk of ovarian cancer is significantly higher in premenarcheal and postmenopausal women with an adnexal mass than in women of reproductive age.

C. Diagnostic workup

1. Initial evaluation with a thorough history, physical examination, and vaginal probe ultrasonography will distinguish most benign masses from malignant masses. Chest X-ray is performed to rule out parenchymal or pleural involvement with effusion. Screening mammography, if it has not been done within 6-12 months, should be performed preoperatively to rule out another primary source.

2. Other studies that may be helpful in the diagnostic workup include barium enema, upper gastrointestinal series, colonoscopy, upper gastrointestinal endoscopy, intravenous pyelography, and computed tomography (CT) scan or magnetic resonance imaging.

3. The tumor marker CA 125 may assist in evaluation. Sustained elevation of CA 125 levels occurs in more than 80% of patients with nonmucinous epithelial ovarian carcinomas but in only 1% of the general population. Levels of CA 125 in serum also may be elevated in patients with conditions such as endometriosis, leiomyomata, pelvic inflammatory disease, hepatitis, congestive heart failure, cirrhosis, and malignancies other than ovarian carcinomas. In postmenopausal patients with pelvic masses, CA 125 levels in serum greater than 65 U/mL are predictive of a malignancy in 75% of cases.

III. Primary treatment of epithelial ovarian cancer

A. Primary therapy for ovarian cancer is complete staging and optimal reduction of tumor volume. Subsequent therapy depends on the operative findings.

B. Staging

1. Ovarian cancer staging is based on surgical evaluation. Accurate staging is of utmost importance for planning further therapy and in discussing prognosis. Staging is determined by clinical, surgical, histologic, and pathologic findings, including results of cytologic testing of effusions or peritoneal washings. Pleural effusions should be sampled.

2. **Operative techniques**

   a. The incision used should provide maximum exposure of the pelvis and allow thorough evaluation of the upper abdomen. If present, ascites should be aspirated and sent for cytopathologic evaluation. A small amount of heparin should be added to prevent clotting of bloody or mucoid specimens. If ascites is not present, abdominal washings with saline should be obtained from the pericolic gutters, the suprahepatic space, and the pelvis. A Pap test of the diaphragm should be taken.

   b. The abdominal cavity should be explored systematically. The lower surface of the diaphragm, the upper abdominal recesses, the liver, and retroperitoneal nodes should be carefully noted for tumor involvement. In addition, the intestines, mesentery, and omentum should be examined. The presence or absence of metastases in the pelvis and abdomen should be noted, and the exact location and size of tumor nodules should be described.

   c. In cases in which disease is grossly confined to the pelvis, efforts should be made to detect occult metastasis with peritoneal cytologies, biopsies of peritoneum from the pelvis and pericolic gutters, and resection of the greater omentum. In addition, selective pelvic and paraaortic lymphadenectomy also should be carried out.

Definitions of the Stages in Primary Carcinoma of the Ovary	
Stage	**Definition**
I	Growth is limited to the ovaries
IA	Growth is limited to one ovary; no ascites present containing malignant cells; no tumor on the external surface; capsule is intact
IB	Growth is limited to both ovaries; no ascites present containing malignant cells; no tumor on the external surfaces; capsules are intact
IC	Tumor is classified as either stage IA or IB but with tumor on the surface of one or both ovaries; or with ruptured capsule(s); or with ascites containing malignant cells present or with positive peritoneal washings
II	Growth involves one or both ovaries with pelvic extension
IIA	Extension and/or metastases to the uterus and/or tubes
IIB	Extension to other pelvic tissues
IIC	Tumor is either stage IIA or IIb but with tumor on the surface of one or both ovaries; or with capsule(s) ruptured; or with ascites containing malignant cells present or with positive peritoneal washings
III	Tumor involves one or both ovaries with peritoneal implants outside the pelvis and/or positive retroperitoneal or inguinal nodes; superficial liver metastasis equals stage III; tumor is limited to the true pelvis but with histologically proven malignant extension to small bowel or omentum
IIIA	Tumor is grossly limited to the true pelvis with negative nodes but with histologically confirmed microscopic seeding of abdominal peritoneal surfaces
IIIB	Tumor involves one or both ovaries with histologically confirmed implants of abdominal peritoneal surfaces, none exceeding 2 cm in diameter; nodes are negative
IIIC	Abdominal implants greater than 2 cm in diameter and/or positive retroperitoneal or inguinal nodes
IV	Growth involves one or both ovaries with distant metastases; if pleural effusion is present, there must be positive cytology findings to assign a case to stage IV; parenchymal liver metastasis equals stage IV

C. **Cytoreductive surgery** improves response to chemotherapy and survival of women with advanced ovarian cancer. Operative management is designed to remove as much tumor as possible. When a malignant tumor is present, a thorough abdominal exploration, total abdominal hysterectomy, bilateral salpingo-oophorectomy, lymphadenectomy, omentectomy, and removal of all gross cancer are standard therapy.

D. **Adjuvant therapy**
   1. Patients with stage IA or IB disease (who have been completely surgically staged) and who have borderline, well- or moderately differentiated tumors do not benefit from additional chemotherapy because their prognosis is excellent with surgery alone.
   2. Chemotherapy improves survival and is an effective means of palliation of ovarian cancer. In patients who are at increased risk of recurrence (stage I G3 and all IC-IV), chemotherapy is recommended. Sequential clinical trials of chemotherapy agents demonstrate that

cisplatin (or carboplatin) given in combination with paclitaxel is the most active combination identified.

References: See page 140.

Obstetrics

Prenatal Care

I. **Prenatal history and physical examination**
   A. **Diagnosis of pregnancy**
      1. **Amenorrhea** is usually the first sign of conception. Other symptoms include breast fullness and tenderness, skin changes, nausea, vomiting, urinary frequency, and fatigue.
      2. **Pregnancy tests.** Urine pregnancy tests may be positive within days of the first missed menstrual period. Serum beta human chorionic gonadotropin (HCG) is accurate up to a few days after implantation.
      3. **Fetal heart tones** can be detected as early as 11-12 weeks from the last menstrual period (LMP) by Doppler. The normal fetal heart rate is 120-160 beats per minute.
      4. **Fetal movements** ("quickening") are first felt by the patient at 17-19 weeks.
      5. **Ultrasound** will visualize a gestational sac at 5-6 weeks and a fetal pole with movement and cardiac activity by 7-8 weeks. Ultrasound can estimate fetal age accurately if completed before 24 weeks.
      6. **Estimated date of confinement.** The mean duration of pregnancy is 40 weeks from the LMP. Estimated date of confinement (EDC) can be calculated by Nägele's rule: Add 7 days to the first day of the LMP, then subtract 3 months.
   B. **Contraceptive history.** Recent oral contraceptive usage often causes postpill amenorrhea, and may cause erroneous pregnancy dating.
   C. **Gynecologic and obstetric history**
      1. Gravidity is the total number of pregnancies. Parity is expressed as the number of term pregnancies, preterm pregnancies, abortions, and live births.
      2. The character and length of previous labors, type of delivery, complications, infant status, and birth weight are recorded.
      3. Assess prior cesarean sections and determine type of C-section (low transverse or classical), and determine reason it was performed.
   D. **Medical and surgical history** and prior hospitalizations are documented.
   E. **Medications** and allergies are recorded.
   F. **Family history** of medical illnesses, hereditary illness, or multiple gestation is sought.
   G. **Social history.** Cigarettes, alcohol, or illicit drug use.
   H. **Review of systems.** Abdominal pain, constipation, headaches, vaginal bleeding, dysuria or urinary frequency, or hemorrhoids.
   I. **Physical examination**
      1. Weight, funduscopic examination, thyroid, breast, lungs, and heart are examined.
      2. An extremity and neurologic exam are completed, and the presence of a cesarean section scar is sought.
      3. **Pelvic examination**
         a. Pap smear and culture for gonorrhea are completed routinely. Chlamydia culture is completed in high-risk patients.
         b. **Estimation of gestational age by uterine size**
            (1) The nongravid uterus is 3 x 4 x 7 cm. The uterus begins to change in size at 5-6 weeks.
            (2) Gestational age is estimated by uterine size: 8 weeks = 2 x normal size; 10 weeks = 3 x normal; 12 weeks = 4 x normal.
            (3) At 12 weeks the fundus becomes palpable at the symphysis pubis.
            (4) At 16 weeks, the uterus is midway between the symphysis pubis and the umbilicus.
            (5) At 20 weeks, the uterus is at the umbilicus. After 20 weeks,

there is a correlation between the number of weeks of gestation and the number of centimeters from the pubic symphysis to the top of the fundus.

(6) Uterine size that exceeds the gestational dating by 3 or more weeks suggests multiple gestation, molar pregnancy, or (most commonly) an inaccurate date for LMP. Ultrasonography will confirm inaccurate dating or intrauterine growth failure.

    c. Adnexa are palpated for masses.

II. Initial visit laboratory testing

A. CBC, AB blood typing and Rh factor, antibody screen, rubella, VDRL/RPR, hepatitis B surface Ag.

B. Pap smear, urine pregnancy test, urinalysis and urine culture. Cervical culture for gonorrhea and chlamydia.

C. Tuberculosis skin testing, HIV counseling/testing.

D. Hemoglobin electrophoresis is indicated in risks groups, such as sickle hemoglobin in African patients, B-thalassemia in Mediterranean patients, and alpha-thalassemia in Asian patients. Tay-Sachs carrier testing is indicated in Jewish patients.

III. Clinical assessment at first trimester prenatal visits

A. Assessment at each prenatal visit includes maternal weight, blood pressure, uterine size, and evaluation for edema, proteinuria, and glucosuria.

B. First Doppler heart tones should become detectable at 10-12 weeks, and they should be sought thereafter.

C. Routine prenatal vitamins are probably not necessary. Folic acid supplementation preconceptually and throughout the early part of pregnancy has been shown to decrease the incidence of fetal neural tube defects.

Frequency of Prenatal Care Visits in Low-Risk Pregnancies	
<28 weeks	Every month
28-36 weeks	Every 2 weeks
36-delivery	Every 1 week until delivery

D. First Trimester Education. Discuss smoking, alcohol, exercise, diet, and sexuality.

E. Headache and backache. Acetaminophen (Tylenol) 325-650 mg every 3-4 hours is effective. Aspirin is contraindicated.

F. Nausea and vomiting. First-trimester morning sickness may be relieved by eating frequent, small meals, getting out of bed slowly after eating a few crackers, and by avoiding spicy or greasy foods. Promethazine (Phenergan) 12.5-50 mg PO q4-6h prn or diphenhydramine (Benadryl) 25-50 mg tid-qid is useful.

G. Constipation. A high-fiber diet with psyllium (Metamucil), increased fluid intake, and regular exercise should be advised. Docusate (Colace) 100 mg bid may provide relief.

IV. Clinical assessment at second trimester visits

A. Questions for each follow-up visit

    1. First detection of fetal movement (quickening) should occur at around 17 weeks in a multigravida and at 19 weeks in a primigravida. **Fetal movement** should be documented at each visit after 17 weeks.

    2. Vaginal bleeding or symptoms of preterm labor should be sought.

B. Fetal heart rate is documented at each visit

C. Maternal serum testing at 15-18 weeks

    1. Triple screen (multiple marker screening). In women under age 35 years, screening for fetal Down syndrome is accomplished with a triple screen. Maternal serum alpha-fetoprotein is elevated in 20-25% of all cases of Down syndrome, and it is elevated in fetal neural tube deficits. Levels of hCG are higher in Down syndrome and levels of

unconjugated estriol are lower in Down syndrome.
2. If levels are abnormal, an ultrasound examination is performed and genetic amniocentesis is offered. The triple screen identifies 60% of Down syndrome cases. Low levels of all three serum analytes identifies 60-75% of all cases of fetal trisomy 18.
D. **At 15-18 weeks, genetic amniocentesis** should be offered to patients ≥35 years old, and it should be offered if a birth defect has occurred in the mother, father, or in previous offspring.
E. **Screening ultrasound** should usually be obtained at 16-18 weeks.
F. **At 24-28 weeks**, a one-hour Glucola (blood glucose measurement 1 hour after 50-gm oral glucose) is obtained to screen for gestational diabetes. Those with a particular risk (eg, previous gestational diabetes or fetal macrosomia), require earlier testing. If the 1 hour test result is greater than 140 mg/dL, a 3-hour glucose tolerance test is necessary.
G. **Second trimester education**. Discomforts include backache, round ligament pain, constipation, and indigestion.

V. **Clinical assessment at third trimester visits**
A. **Fetal movement** is documented. Vaginal bleeding or symptoms of preterm labor should be sought. Pregnancy induced hypertension symptoms (blurred vision, headache, rapid weight gain, edema) are sought.
B. **Fetal heart rate** is documented at each visit.
C. **At 26-30 weeks**, repeat hemoglobin and hematocrit are obtained to determine the need for iron supplementation.
D. **At 28-30 weeks**, an antibody screen is obtained in Rh-negative women, and D immune globulin (RhoGAM) is administered if negative.
E. **At 36 weeks**, repeat serologic testing for syphilis is recommended for high risk groups.
F. **Gonorrhea and chlamydia screening is repeated** in the third-trimester in high-risk patients.
G. **Screening for group B streptococcus colonization at 35-37 weeks**
1. Lower vaginal and rectal cultures are recommended; cultures should not be collected by speculum examination. The optimal method for GBS screening is collection of a single standard culture swab of the distal vagina and anorectum.
H. **Third trimester education**
1. **Signs of labor.** The patient should call physician when rupture of membranes or contractions have occurred every 5 minutes for one hour.
2. **Danger signs.** Preterm labor, rupture of membranes, bleeding, edema, signs of preeclampsia.
3. **Common discomforts.** Cramps, edema, frequent urination.
I. **At 36 weeks**, a cervical exam may be completed. Fetal position should be assessed by palpation (Leopold's Maneuvers).
References: See page 140.

Normal Labor

Labor consists of the process by which uterine contractions expel the fetus. A term pregnancy is 37 to 42 weeks from the last menstrual period (LMP).
I. **Obstetrical History and Physical Examination**
A. **History of the present labor**
1. **Contractions.** The frequency, duration, onset, and intensity of uterine contractions should be determined. Contractions may be accompanied by a "bloody show" (passage of blood-tinged mucus from the dilating cervical os). Braxton Hicks contractions are often felt by patients during the last weeks of pregnancy. They are usually irregular, mild, and do not cause cervical change.
2. **Rupture of membranes.** Leakage of fluid may occur alone or in conjunction with uterine contractions. The patient may report a large

gush of fluid or increased moisture. The color of the liquid should be determine, including the presence of blood or meconium.

3. **Vaginal bleeding** should be assessed. Spotting or blood-tinged mucus is common in normal labor. Heavy vaginal bleeding may be a sign of placental abruption.

4. **Fetal movement.** A progressive decrease in fetal movement from baseline, should prompt an assessment of fetal well-being with a nonstress test or biophysical profile.

B. **History of present pregnancy**
1. **Estimated date of confinement** (EDC) is calculated as 40 weeks from the first day of the LMP.
2. **Fetal heart tones** are first heard with a Doppler instrument 10-12 weeks from the LMP.
3. **Quickening** (maternal perception of fetal movement) occurs at about 17 weeks.
4. **Uterine size** before 16 weeks is an accurate measure of dates.
5. **Ultrasound** measurement of fetal size before 24 weeks of gestation is an accurate measure of dates.
6. **Prenatal history**. Medical problems during this pregnancy should be reviewed, including urinary tract infections, diabetes, or hypertension.
7. **Review of systems.** Severe headaches, scotomas, hand and facial edema, or epigastric pain (preeclampsia) should be sought. Dysuria, urinary frequency or flank pain may indicate cystitis or pyelonephritis.

C. **Obstetrical history.** Past pregnancies, durations and outcomes, preterm deliveries, operative deliveries, prolonged labors, pregnancy-induced hypertension should be assessed.

D. **Past medical history** of asthma, hypertension, or renal disease should be sought.

II. **Physical Examination**
A. Vital signs are assessed.
B. **Head.** Funduscopy should seek hemorrhages or exudates, which may suggest diabetes or hypertension. Facial, hand and ankle edema suggest preeclampsia.
C. **Chest.** Auscultation of the lungs for wheezes and crackles may indicate asthma or heart failure.
D. **Uterine Size.** Until the middle of the third trimester, the distance in centimeters from the pubic symphysis to the uterine fundus should correlate with the gestational age in weeks. Toward term, the measurement becomes progressively less reliable because of engagement of the presenting part.
E. **Estimation of fetal weight** is completed by palpation of the gravid uterus.
F. **Leopold's maneuvers** are used to determine the position of the fetus.
1. **The first maneuver** determines which fetal pole occupies the uterine fundus. The breech moves with the fetal body. The vertex is rounder and harder, feels more globular than the breech, and can be moved separately from the fetal body.
2. **Second maneuver.** The lateral aspects of the uterus are palpated to determine on which side the fetal back or fetal extremities (the small parts) are located.
3. **Third maneuver.** The presenting part is moved from side to side. If movement is difficult, engagement of the presenting part has occurred.
4. **Fourth maneuver.** With the fetus presenting by vertex, the cephalic prominence may be palpable on the side of the fetal small parts.
G. **Pelvic examination.** The adequacy of the bony pelvis, the integrity of the fetal membranes, the degree of cervical dilatation and effacement, and the station of the presenting part should be determined.
H. **Extremities.** Severe lower extremity or hand edema suggests preeclampsia. Deep-tendon hyperreflexia and clonus may signal impending seizures.
I. **Laboratory tests**
1. Prenatal labs should be documented, including CBC, blood type, Rh, antibody screen, serologic test for syphilis, rubella antibody titer,

urinalysis, culture, Pap smear, cervical cultures for gonorrhea and Chlamydia, and hepatitis B surface antigen (HbsAg).
2. During labor, the CBC, urinalysis and RPR are repeated. The HBSAG is repeated for high-risk patients. A clot of blood is placed on hold.
J. Fetal heart rate. The baseline heart rate, variability, accelerations, and decelerations are recorded.

Labor History and Physical

Chief compliant: Contractions, rupture of membranes.
HPI: ___ year old Gravida (number of pregnancies) Para (number of deliveries).
Gestational age, last menstrual period, estimated date of confinement.
Contractions (onset, frequency, intensity), rupture of membranes (time, color). Vaginal bleeding (consistency, quantity, bloody show); fetal movement.
Fetal Heart Rate Strip: Baseline rate, accelerations, reactivity, decelerations, contraction frequency.
Dates: First day of last menstrual period, estimated date of confinement. Ultrasound dating.
Prenatal Care: Date of first exam, number of visits; has size been equal to dates? infections, hypertension, diabetes.
Obstetrical History: Dates of prior pregnancies, gestational age, route (C-section with indications and type of uterine incision), weight, complications, length of labor, hypertension.
Gynecologic History: Menstrual history (menarche, interval, duration), herpes, gonorrhea, chlamydia, abortions; oral contraceptives.
Past Medical History: Illnesses, asthma, hypertension, diabetes, renal disease, surgeries.
Medications: Iron, prenatal vitamins.
Allergies: Penicillin, codeine?
Social History: Smoking, alcohol, drug use.
Family History: Hypertension, diabetes, bleeding disorders.
Review of Systems: Severe headaches, scotomas, blurred vision, hand and face edema, epigastric pain, pruritus, dysuria, fever.

Physical Exam
General Appearance:
Vitals: BP, pulse, respirations, temperature.
HEENT: Funduscopy, facial edema, jugular venous distention.
Chest: Wheezes, rhonchi.
Cardiovascular: Rhythm, S1, S2, murmurs.
Abdomen: Fundal height, Leopold's maneuvers (lie, presentation). Estimated fetal weight (EFW), tenderness, scars.
Cervix: Dilatation, effacement, station, position, status of membranes, presentation. Vulvar herpes lesions.
Extremities: Cyanosis, clubbing, edema.
Neurologic: Deep tender reflexes, clonus.
Prenatal Labs: Obtain results of one hour post glucola, RPR/VDRL, rubella, blood type, Rh, CBC, Pap, PPD, hepatitis BsAg, UA, C and S.
Current Labs: Hemoglobin, hematocrit, glucose, UA; urine dipstick for protein.
Assessment: Intrauterine pregnancy (IUP) at 40 weeks, admitted with the following problems:
Plan: Anticipated type of labor and delivery. List plan for each problem.

III. **Normal labor**
   A. Labor is characterized by uterine contractions of sufficient frequency, intensity, and duration to result in effacement and dilatation of the cervix.
   B. **The first stage of labor** starts with the onset of regular contractions and ends with complete dilatation (10 cm). This stage is further subdivided into the latent and an active phases.
      1. The latent phase starts with the onset of regular uterine contractions and is characterized by slow cervical dilatation to 4 cm. The latent phase is variable in length.
      2. The active phase follows and is characterized by more rapid dilatation to 10 cm. During the active phase of labor, the average rate of cervical dilatation is 1.5 cm/hour in the multipara and 1.2 cm/hour in the nullipara.
   C. **The second stage of labor** begins with complete dilatation of the cervix and ends with delivery of the infant. It is characterized by voluntary and involuntary pushing. The average second stage of labor is one-half hour in a multipara and 1 hour in the primipara.
   D. **The third stage of labor** begins with the delivery of the infant and ends with the delivery of the placenta.
   E. **Intravenous fluids**. IV fluid during labor is usually Ringer's lactate or 0.45% normal saline with 5% dextrose. Intravenous fluid infused rapidly or given as a bolus should be dextrose-free because maternal hyperglycemia can occur.
   F. **Activity.** Patients in the latent phase of labor are usually allowed to walk.
   G. **Narcotic and analgesic drugs**
      1. Nalbuphine (Nubain) 5 to 10 mg SC or IV q2-3h.
      2. Butorphanol (Stadol) 2 mg IM q3-4h or 0.5-1.0 mg IV q1.5-2.0h **OR**
      3. Meperidine (Demerol) 50 to 100 mg IM q3-4h or 10 to 25 mg IV q1.5-3.0 h **OR**
      4. Narcotics should be avoided if their peak action will not have diminished by the time of delivery. Respiratory depression is reversed with naloxone (Narcan): Adults, 0.4 mg IV or IM and neonates, 0.01 mg/kg.
   H. **Epidural anesthesia**
      1. Contraindications include infection in the lumbar area, clotting defect, active neurologic disease, sensitivity to the anesthetic, hypovolemia, and septicemia.
      2. Risks include hypotension, respiratory arrest, toxic drug reaction, and rare neurologic complications. An epidural has no significant effect on the progress of labor.
      3. Before the epidural is initiated, the patient is hydrated with 500-1000 mL of dextrose-free intravenous fluid.

Labor and Delivery Admitting Orders

Admit: Labor and Delivery
Diagnoses: Intrauterine pregnancy at _____ weeks.
Condition: Satisfactory
Vitals: q1 hr per routine
Activity: May ambulate as tolerated.
Nursing: I and O. Catheterize prn; external or internal monitors.
Diet: NPO except ice chips.
IV Fluids: Lactated Ringers with 5% dextrose at 125 cc/h.
Medications:
Epidural at 4-5 cm.
Nalbuphine (Nubain) 5-10 mg IV/SC q2-3h prn **OR**
Butorphanol (Stadol) 0.5-1 mg IV q1.5-2h prn **OR**
Meperidine (Demerol) 25-75 mg slow IV q1.5-3h prn pain **AND**
Promethazine (Phenergan) 25-50 mg, IV q3-4h prn nausea **OR**
Hydroxyzine (Vistaril) 25-50 mg IV q3-4h prn
Fleet enema PR prn constipation.
Labs: CBC, dipstick urine protein, blood type and Rh, antibody screen, VDRL, HBSAG, rubella, type and screen (C-section).

I. **Intrapartum chemoprophylaxis for group B streptococcus infection**
   1. Intrapartum chemoprophylaxis is offered to all pregnant women identified as GBS carriers by a culture obtained at 35-37 weeks.
   2. If the result of GBS culture is not known at the time of labor, intrapartum chemoprophylaxis should be administered if one of the following is present: Gestation <37 weeks, duration of membrane rupture ≥18 hours, or temperature ≥38°C (100.4°F).
   3. Women found to have GBS bacteriuria during pregnancy should be treated at the time of diagnosis, and they should receive intrapartum chemoprophylaxis. Intrapartum chemoprophylaxis should be given to women with a history of previously giving birth to an infant with GBS disease.
   4. Intrapartum chemoprophylaxis consists of penicillin G, 5 million units, then 2.5 million units IV every 4 hours until delivery. Ampicillin, 2 g initially and then 1 g IV every 4 hours until delivery, is an alternative. Clindamycin or erythromycin may be used for women allergic to penicillin.

IV. **Normal spontaneous vaginal delivery**
   A. **Preparation.** As the multiparous patient approaches complete dilatation or as the nulliparous patient begins to crown the fetal scalp, preparations are made for delivery.
   B. **Maternal position.** The mother is usually placed in the dorsal lithotomy position with left lateral tilt.
   C. **Delivery of a fetus in an occiput anterior position**
      1. **Delivery of the head**
         a. The fetal head is delivered by extension as the flexed head passes through the vaginal introitus.
         b. Once the fetal head has been delivered, external rotation to the occiput transverse position occurs.
         c. The oropharynx and nose of the fetus are suctioned with the bulb syringe. A finger is passed into the vagina along the fetal neck to check for a nuchal cord. If one is present, it is lifted over the vertex. If this cannot be accomplished, the cord is doubly clamped and divided.
         d. If shoulder dystocia is anticipated, the shoulders should be delivered immediately.
      2. **Episiotomy** consists of incision of the perineum, enlarging the vaginal

orifice at the time of delivery. If indicated, an episiotomy should be performed when 3-4 cm of fetal scalp is visible.

a. With adequate local or spinal anesthetic in place, a medial episiotomy is completed by incising the perineum toward the anus and into the vagina.

b. Avoid cutting into the anal sphincter or the rectum. A short perineum may require a mediolateral episiotomy.

c. Application of pressure at the perineal apex with a towel-covered hand helps to prevent extension of the episiotomy.

3. **Delivery of the anterior shoulder** is accomplished by gentle downward traction on the fetal head. The posterior shoulder is delivered by upward traction.

4. **Delivery of the body.** The infant is grasped around the back with the left hand, and the right hand is placed, near the vagina, under the baby's buttocks, supporting the infant's body. The infant's body is rotated toward the operator and supported by the operator's forearm, freeing the right hand to suction the mouth and nose. The baby's head should be kept lower than the body to facilitate drainage of secretions.

5. **Suctioning** of the nose and oropharynx is repeated.

6. **The umbilical cord** is doubly clamped and cut, leaving 2-3 cm of cord.

D. Delivery of the placenta

1. The placenta usually separates spontaneously from the uterine wall within 5 minutes of delivery. Gentle fundal massage and gentle traction on the cord facilitates delivery of the placenta.

2. The placenta should be examined for missing cotyledons or blind vessels. The cut end of the cord should be examined for 2 arteries and a vein. The absence of one umbilical artery suggests a congenital anomaly.

3. Prophylaxis against excessive postpartum blood loss consists of external fundal massage and oxytocin (Pitocin), 20 units in 1000 mL of IV fluid at 100 drops/minute after delivery of the placenta. Oxytocin can cause marked hypotension if administered as a IV bolus.

4. After delivery of the placenta, the birth canal is inspected for lacerations.

Delivery Note

1. Note the age, gravida, para, and gestational age.
2. Time of birth, type of birth (spontaneous vaginal delivery), position (left occiput anterior).
3. Bulb suctioned, sex, weight, APGAR scores, nuchal cord, and number of cord vessels.
4. Placenta expressed spontaneously intact. Describe episiotomy degree and repair technique.
5. Note lacerations of cervix, vagina, rectum, perineum.
6. Estimated blood loss:
7. Disposition: Mother to recovery room in stable condition. Infant to nursery in stable condition.

Routine Postpartum Orders

Transfer: To recovery room, then postpartum ward when stable.
Vitals: Check vitals, bleeding, fundus q15min x 1 hr or until stable, then q4h.
Activity: Ambulate in 2 hours if stable
Nursing Orders: If unable to void, straight catheterize; sitz baths prn with 1:1000 Betadine prn, ice pack to perineum prn, record urine output.
Diet: Regular
IV Fluids: D5LR at 125 cc/h. Discontinue when stable and taking PO diet.
Medications:
    Oxytocin (Pitocin) 20 units in 1 L D5LR at 100 drops/minute or 10 U IM.
    FeSO4 325 mg PO bid-tid.
Symptomatic Medications:
    Acetaminophen/codeine (Tylenol #3) 1-2 tab PO q3-4h prn **OR**
    Oxycodone/acetaminophen (Percocet) 1 tab q6h prn pain.
    Milk of magnesia 30 mL PO q6h prn constipation.
    Docusate Sodium (Colace) 100 mg PO bid.
    Dulcolax suppository PR prn constipation.
    A and D cream or Lanolin prn if breast feeding.
    Breast binder or tight brazier and ice packs prn if not to breast feed.
Labs: Hemoglobin/hematocrit in AM. Give rubella vaccine if titer <1:10.

Classification and Repair of Perineal Lacerations and Episiotomies

I. **First-degree laceration**
    A. A first degree perineal laceration extends only through the vaginal and perineal skin.
    B. **Repair:** Place a single layer of interrupted 3-O chromic or Vicryl sutures about 1 cm apart.
II. **Second-degree laceration and repair of midline episiotomy**
    A. A second degree laceration extends deeply into the soft tissues of the perineum, down to, but not including, the external anal sphincter capsule. The disruption involves the bulbocavernosus and transverse perineal muscles.
    B. **Repair**
        1. Proximate the deep tissues of the perineal body by placing 3-4 interrupted 2-O or 3-O chromic or Vicryl absorbable sutures. Reapproximate the superficial layers of the perineal body with a running suture extending to the bottom of the episiotomy.
        2. Identify the apex of the vaginal laceration. Suture the vaginal mucosa with running, interlocking, 3-O chromic or Vicryl absorbable suture.
        3. Close the perineal skin with a running, subcuticular suture. Tie off the suture and remove the needle.
III. **Third-degree laceration**
    A. This laceration extends through the perineum and through the anal sphincter.

   B. Repair
      1. Identify each severed end of the external anal sphincter capsule, and grasp each end with an Allis clamp.
      2. Proximate the capsule with the sphincter with 4 interrupted sutures of 2-O or 3-O Vicryl suture, making sure the sutures do not penetrate the rectal mucosa.
      3. Continue the repair as for a second degree laceration as above. Stool softeners and sitz baths are prescribed post-partum.

IV. **Fourth-degree laceration**
   A. The laceration extends through the perineum, anal sphincter, and extends through the rectal mucosa to expose the lumen of the rectum.
   B. **Repair**
      1. Irrigate the laceration with sterile saline solution. Identify the anatomy, including the apex of the rectal mucosal laceration.
      2. Approximate the rectal submucosa with a running suture using a 3-O chromic on a GI needle extending to the margin of the anal skin.
      3. Place a second layer of running suture to invert the first suture line, and take some tension from the first layer closure.
      4. Identify and grasp the torn edges of the external anal sphincter capsule with Allis clamps, and perform a repair as for a third-degree laceration. Close the remaining layers as for a second-degree laceration.
      5. A low-residue diet, stool softeners, and sitz baths are prescribed post-partum.

References: See page 140.

Fetal Heart Rate Monitoring

Intrapartum fetal heart rate (FHR) monitoring can detect fetal hypoxia, umbilical cord compression, tachycardia, and acidosis. Fetal heart rate monitoring can significantly reduce the risk of newborn seizures (relative risk 0.5).

I. **Pathophysiology**
   A. Uterine contractions decrease placental blood flow and result in intermittent episodes of decreased oxygen delivery.
   B. The fetus normally tolerates contractions without difficulty, but if the frequency, duration, or strength of contractions becomes excessive, fetal hypoxemia may result.

II. **Fetal heart rate monitoring method**
   A. Continuous FHR and contraction monitoring may be accomplished externally or internally. Internal FHR monitoring is accomplished with a spiral wire attached to the fetal scalp or other presenting part.
   B. Uterine contractions are monitored externally or internally. The paper speed is usually 3 cm/min.

III. **Fetal heart rate patterns**
   A. **Fetal heart rate**
      1. The FHR at term ranges from 120-160 bpm. The initial response of the FHR to intermittent hypoxia is deceleration, but tachycardia may develop if the hypoxia is prolonged and severe.
      2. Tachycardia may also be associated with maternal fever, intra-amniotic infection, and congenital heart disease.
   B. **Fetal heart rate variability**
      1. Decreasing fetal heart rate variability is a fetal response to hypoxia. Fetal sleep cycles or medications may also decrease the FHR variability.
      2. The development of decreased variability in the absence of decelerations is unlikely to be due to hypoxia.
   C. **Accelerations**
      1. Accelerations are common periodic changes, which are usually associated with fetal movement.
      2. These changes are reassuring and almost always confirm that the fetus is not acidotic.

D. Variable decelerations

1. Variable decelerations are characterized by slowing of the FHR with an abrupt onset and return. They are frequently followed by small accelerations of the FHR. These decelerations vary in depth, duration, and shape. Variable decelerations are associated with cord compression, and they usually coincide with the timing of the uterine contractions.
2. Variable decelerations are caused by umbilical cord compression, and they are the most common decelerations seen in labor. These decelerations are generally associated with a favorable outcome. Persistent, deep, and long lasting variable decelerations are nonreassuring.
3. Persistent variable decelerations to less than 70 bpm lasting more than 60 seconds are concerning.
4. Variable decelerations with a persistently slow return to baseline are nonreassuring because they reflect persistent hypoxia. Nonreassuring variable decelerations are associated with tachycardia, absence of accelerations, and loss of variability.

E. Late decelerations

1. Late decelerations are U-shaped with a gradual onset and gradual return. They are usually shallow (10-30 beats per minute), and they reach their nadir after the peak of the contraction.
2. Late decelerations occur when uterine contractions cause decreased fetal oxygenation. In milder cases, they can be a result of CNS hypoxia. In more severe cases, they may be the result of direct myocardial depression.
3. Late decelerations become deeper as the degree of hypoxia becomes more severe. Occasional or intermittent late decelerations are not uncommon during labor. When late decelerations become persistent, they are nonreassuring.

F. Early decelerations

1. Early decelerations are shallow and symmetrical with a pattern similar to that of late decelerations, but they reach their nadir at the same time as the peak of the contraction.
2. These decelerations occur in the active phase of labor and are benign changes caused by fetal head compression.

G. **Prolonged decelerations** are isolated, abrupt decreases in the FHR to levels below baseline, for at least 60-90 seconds.

1. These changes may be caused by fetal hypoxia.
2. The degree to which such decelerations are nonreassuring depends on their depth and duration, loss of variability, and the frequency and progression of recurrence.

IV. Management of nonreassuring patterns

A. Approach to nonreassuring patterns

1. Determine the etiology of the pattern.
2. Attempt to correct the pattern by correcting the primary problem or by instituting measures aimed at improving fetal oxygenation and placental perfusion.
3. If attempts to correct the pattern are not successful, a scalp or sound stimulation test or fetal scalp blood pH assessment should be considered.
4. The need for operative intervention should be assessed.

B. Late decelerations. Excessive uterine contractions, maternal hypotension, or maternal hypoxemia should be corrected.

C. Severe variable or prolonged decelerations

1. A pelvic examination is performed to rule out umbilical cord prolapse or rapid descent of the fetal head.
2. If no causes are found, umbilical cord compression is likely to be responsible.

D. Measures that improve fetal oxygenation and placental perfusion

1. **Oxygen therapy.** Maternal oxygenation may be increased by giving oxygen at a flow rate of 8-10 L/min with a tight-fitting face mask.

2. **Maternal position**
   a. In the supine position, the vena cava and aortoiliac vessels are compressed by the gravid uterus. This results in decreased return of blood to the maternal heart, leading to a fall in uterine blood flow.
   b. **The lateral recumbent position** (either side) is best for maximizing cardiac output and uterine blood flow, and it is often associated with an improvement in the FHR.
3. **Oxytocin (Pitocin).** If nonreassuring FHR changes occur in patients receiving oxytocin, the infusion should be discontinued. Restarting the infusion at a lower rate may be better tolerated.
4. **Intravenous hydration.** If the mother is hypovolemic, intravenous hydration should be initiated.
5. **Amnioinfusion**
   a. Variable decelerations that occur prior to fetal descent at 8-9 cm of dilatation are most frequently caused by oligohydramnios. Replacement of amniotic fluid with normal saline infused through an intrauterine pressure catheter decreases variable decelerations in patients with decreased amniotic fluid volume.
   b. Saline amnioinfusion also decreases newborn respiratory complications from meconium due to the dilutional effect of amnioinfusion.
   c. Continuous amnioinfusion begins with a loading dose of 10 mL/min for 1 hour, followed by a maintenance dose of 3 mL/min via a double-lumen uterine pressure catheter.
6. **Tocolytic agents**
   a. If a nonreassuring FHR pattern results from excessive uterine contractions, uterine activity can be decreased with tocolytics.
   b. Terbutaline, 0.25 mg subcutaneously or 0.125-0.25 mg intravenously, will suppress contractions. Magnesium sulfate is also of value in providing rapid uterine relaxation.
   c. Even in the absence of excessive uterine contractions, newborn condition may be improved by tocolytic agents.

V. **Management of persistent nonreassuring fetal heart rate patterns**
   A. **Persistent nonreassuring decelerations with normal FHR variability and absence of tachycardia** generally indicate a lack of fetal acidosis.
   B. **Persistent late decelerations or severe variable decelerations associated with absence of variability** are nonreassuring and generally require prompt intervention unless they spontaneously resolve or can be corrected rapidly with conservative measures (oxygen, hydration, maternal repositioning). In the presence of nonreassuring decelerations, a fetal scalp electrode should be placed.
   C. **Spontaneous accelerations** of greater than 15 bpm, lasting at least 15 seconds indicate the absence of fetal acidosis. Fetal scalp stimulation or vibroacoustic stimulation can be used to induce accelerations. If the fetus fails to respond to stimulation in the presence of an otherwise nonreassuring pattern, there is a 50% chance of acidosis.
   D. In cases in which the FHR patterns are persistently nonreassuring, the fetus should be delivered by either cesarean section or rapid vaginal delivery.

Management of Variant Fetal Heart Rate Patterns		
FHR Pattern	**Diagnosis**	**Action**
Normal rate normal variability, accelerations, no decelerations	Fetus is well oxygenated	None

FHR Pattern	Diagnosis	Action
Normal variability, accelerations, mild variant pattern (bradycardia, late decelerations, variable decelerations)	Fetus is still well oxygenated centrally	Conservative management. This is a variant pattern
Normal variability, ± accelerations, moderate-severe variant pattern (bradycardia, late decelerations, variable decelerations)	Fetus is still well oxygenated centrally, but the FHR suggests hypoxia	Continue conservative management. Consider amnioinfusion and/or stimulation testing. Prepare for rapid delivery if pattern worsens
Decreasing variability, ± accelerations, moderate-severe variant patterns (bradycardia, late decelerations, variable decelerations)	Fetus may be on the verge of decompensation	Deliver if spontaneous delivery is remote, or if stimulation supports diagnosis of decompensation. Normal response to stimulation may allow time to await a vaginal delivery
Absent variability, no accelerations, moderate/severe variant patterns (bradycardia, late decelerations, variable decelerations)	Evidence of actual or impending asphyxia	Deliver. Stimulation or in-utero management may be attempted if delivery is not delayed

References: See page 140.

Antepartum Fetal Surveillance

Antepartum fetal surveillance techniques are now routinely used to assess the risk of fetal death in pregnancies complicated by preexisting maternal conditions (eg, type 1 diabetes mellitus) as well as those in which complications have developed (eg, intrauterine growth restriction).

I. Antepartum fetal surveillance techniques
   A. Fetal movement assessment ("kick counts")
      1. A diminution in the maternal perception of fetal movement often but not invariably precedes fetal death, in some cases by several days.
      2. The woman lies on her side and counts distinct fetal movements. Perception of 10 distinct movements in a period of up to 2 hours is considered reassuring. Once 10 movements have been perceived, the count may be discontinued. In the absence of a reassuring count, further fetal assessment is recommended.
   B. Contraction stress test
      1. The CST is based on the response of the fetal heart rate to uterine contractions. It relies on the premise that fetal oxygenation will be transiently worsened by uterine contractions. In the suboptimally oxygenated fetus, the resultant intermittent worsening in oxygenation will, in turn, lead to the fetal heart rate pattern of late decelerations. Uterine contractions also may provoke or accentuate a pattern of variable decelerations caused by fetal umbilical cord compression, which in some cases is associated with oligohydramnios.
      2. With the patient in the lateral recumbent position, the fetal heart rate and uterine contractions are simultaneously recorded with an external

fetal monitor. If at least three spontaneous contractions of 40 seconds' duration each or longer are present in a 10-minute period, no uterine stimulation is necessary. If fewer than three contractions of at least 40 seconds' duration occur in 10 minutes, contractions are induced with either nipple stimulation or intravenous administration of dilute oxytocin. An intravenous infusion of dilute oxytocin may be initiated at a rate of 0.5 mU/min and doubled every 20 minutes until an adequate contraction pattern is achieved.

3. The CST is interpreted according to the presence or absence of late fetal heart rate decelerations, which are defined as decelerations that reach their nadir after the peak of the contraction and that usually persist beyond the end of the contraction. The results of the CST are categorized as follows:
   a. **Negative:** no late or significant variable decelerations
   b. **Positive:** late decelerations following 50% or more of contractions (even if the contraction frequency is fewer than three in 10 minutes)
   c. **Equivocal-suspicious:** intermittent late decelerations or significant variable decelerations
   d. **Equivocal-hyperstimulatory:** fetal heart rate decelerations that occur in the presence of contractions more frequent than every 2 minutes or lasting longer than 90 seconds
   e. **Unsatisfactory:** fewer than three contractions in 10 minutes or an uninterpretable tracing
4. **Relative contraindications to the CST:**
   a. Preterm labor or certain patients at high risk of pre-term labor
   b. Preterm membrane rupture
   c. History of extensive uterine surgery or classical cesarean delivery
   d. Known placenta previa

C. **Nonstress test**
1. The NST is based on the premise that the heart rate of the fetus that is not acidotic or neurologically depressed will temporarily accelerate with fetal movement. Heart rate reactivity is a good indicator of normal fetal autonomic function. Loss of reactivity is associated most commonly with a fetal sleep cycle but may result from any cause of central nervous system depression, including fetal acidosis.
2. With the patient in the lateral tilt position, the fetal heart rate is monitored. The tracing is observed for fetal heart rate accelerations that peak at least 15 beats per minute above the baseline and last 15 seconds from baseline to baseline. Acoustic stimulation of the nonacidotic fetus may elicit fetal heart rate accelerations.
3. The NST is considered reactive (normal) if there are two or more fetal heart rate accelerations (as defined previously) within a 20-minute period, with or without fetal movement discernible by the woman. A nonreactive NST is one that lacks sufficient fetal heart rate accelerations over a 40-minute period. The NST of the noncompromised preterm fetus is frequently nonreactive: from 24 to 28 weeks of gestation, up to 50% of NSTs may not be reactive, and from 28 to 32 weeks of gestation, 15% of NSTs are not reactive.
4. Variable decelerations may be observed in up to 50% of NSTs. If nonrepetitive and brief (<30 seconds), they indicate neither fetal compromise nor the need for obstetric intervention. Repetitive variable decelerations (at least 3 in 20 minutes), even if mild, are associated with an increased risk of cesarean delivery for a nonreassuring intrapartum fetal heart rate pattern. Fetal heart rate decelerations during an NST that persist for 1 minute or longer are associated with a markedly increased risk of both cesarean delivery for a nonreassuring fetal heart rate pattern and fetal demise.

D. **Biophysical profile**
1. The BPP consists of an NST combined with four observations made by ultrasonography. Thus, the BPP comprises five components:
   a. Nonstress test (which, if all four ultrasound components are

normal, may be omitted without compromising the validity of the test results).
   b. Fetal breathing movements (one or more episodes of rhythmic fetal breathing movements of 30 seconds or more within 30 minutes).
   c. Fetal movement (three or more discrete body or limb movements within 30 minutes).
   d. Fetal tone (one or more episodes of extension of a fetal extremity with return to flexion, or opening or closing of a hand).
   e. Determination of the amniotic fluid volume (a single vertical pocket of amniotic fluid exceeding 2 cm is considered evidence of adequate amniotic fluid).

2. Each of the five components is assigned a score of either 2 (normal or present as defined previously) or 0 (abnormal, absent, or insufficient). A composite score of 8 or 10 is normal, a score of 6 is considered equivocal, and a score of 4 or less is abnormal. Regardless of the composite score, in the presence of oligohydramnios (largest vertical pocket of amniotic fluid volume ≤2 cm), further evaluation is warranted.

Components of the Biophysical Profile		
Parameter	Normal (score = 2)	Abnormal (score = 0)
Nonstress test	≥2 accelerations ≥15 beats per minute above baseline during test lasting ≥15 seconds in 20 minutes	<2 accelerations
Amniotic fluid volume	Amniotic fluid index >5 or at least 1 pocket measuring 2 cm x 2 cm in perpendicular planes	AFI <5 or no pocket >2 cm x 2 cm
Fetal breathing movement	Sustained FBM (≥30 seconds)	Absence of FBM or short gasps only <30 seconds total
Fetal body movements	≥3 episodes of either limb or trunk movement	<3 episodes during test
Fetal tone	Extremities in flexion at rest and ≥1 episode of extension of extremity, hand or spine with return to flexion	Extension at rest or no return to flexion after movement

A total score of 8 to 10 is reassuring; a score of 6 is suspicious, and a score of 4 or less is ominous.
Amniotic fluid index = the sum of the largest vertical pocket in each of four quadrants on the maternal abdomen intersecting at the umbilicus.

E. **Modified biophysical profile** combines the NST with the amniotic fluid index (AFI), which is the sum of measurements of the deepest cord-free amniotic fluid pocket in each of the abdominal quadrants, as an indicator of long-term placental function. The modified BPP is considered normal if the NST is reactive and the AFI is more than 5, and abnormal if either the NST is nonreactive or the AFI is 5 or less.

F. **Umbilical artery Doppler velocimetry**
   1. Umbilical artery Doppler flow velocimetry is a technique of fetal surveillance based on the observation that flow velocity waveforms in the umbilical artery of normally growing fetuses differ from those of growth-restricted fetuses. The umbilical flow velocity waveform of normally growing fetuses is characterized by high-velocity diastolic flow, whereas with intrauterine growth restriction, there is diminution of

umbilical artery diastolic flow. Abnormal flow velocity waveforms have been correlated with fetal hypoxia and acidosis and perinatal morbidity and mortality.

2. No benefit has been demonstrated for umbilical artery velocimetry for conditions other than suspected intrauterine growth restriction, such as postterm gestation, diabetes mellitus, systemic lupus erythematosus, or antiphospholipid syndrome. Doppler ultrasonography has not been shown to be of value as a screening test for detecting fetal compromise in the general obstetric population.

II. Clinical considerations and recommendations

A. Indications for antepartum fetal surveillance

1. **Maternal conditions**
   a. Antiphospholipid syndrome
   b. Hyperthyroidism (poorly controlled)
   c. Hemoglobinopathies (hemoglobin SS, SC, or S-thalassemia)
   d. Cyanotic heart disease
   e. Systemic lupus erythematosus
   f. Chronic renal disease
   g. Type 1 diabetes mellitus
   h. Hypertensive disorders

2. **Pregnancy-related conditions**
   a. Pregnancy-induced hypertension
   b. Decreased fetal movement
   c. Oligohydramnios
   d. Polyhydramnios
   e. Intrauterine growth restriction
   f. Postterm pregnancy
   g. Isoimmunization (moderate to severe)
   h. Previous fetal demise (unexplained or recurrent risk)
   i. Multiple gestation (with significant growth discrepancy)

B. Initiation of antepartum fetal surveillance
at 32-34 weeks of gestation is appropriate for most at-risk patients. However, in pregnancies with multiple or particularly worrisome high-risk conditions (eg, chronic hypertension with suspected intrauterine growth restriction), testing might begin as early as 26-28 weeks of gestation.

C. Frequency of testing.
If the maternal medical condition is stable and CST results are negative, the CST is typically repeated in 1 week. Other tests of fetal well-being (NST, BPP, or modified BPP) are typically repeated at weekly intervals, but in the presence of certain high-risk conditions, such as postterm pregnancy, type 1 diabetes, intrauterine growth restriction, or pregnancy-induced hypertension, NST, BPP, or modified BPP testing are performed twice weekly.

Guidelines for Antepartum Testing		
Indication	**Initiation**	**Frequency**
Post-term pregnancy	41 weeks	Twice a week
Preterm rupture of the membranes	At onset	Daily
Bleeding	26 weeks or at onset	Twice a week
Oligohydramnios	26 weeks or at onset	Twice a week
Polyhydramnios	32 weeks	Weekly
Diabetes	32 weeks	Twice a week

Indication	Initiation	Frequency
Chronic or pregnancy-induced hypertension	28 weeks	Weekly. Increase to twice-weekly at 32 weeks.
Steroid-dependent or poorly controlled asthma	28 weeks	Weekly
Sickle cell disease	32 weeks (earlier if symptoms)	Weekly (more often if severe)
Impaired renal function	28 weeks	Weekly
Substance abuse	32 weeks	Weekly
Prior stillbirth	At 2 weeks before prior fetal death	Weekly
Multiple gestation	32 weeks	Weekly
Congenital anomaly	32 weeks	Weekly
Fetal growth restriction	26 weeks	Twice a week or at onset
Decreased fetal movement	At time of complaint	Once

D. **Management of abnormal test results**
   1. Maternal reports of decreased fetal movement should be evaluated by an NST, CST, BPP, or modified BPP; these results, if normal, usually are sufficient to exclude imminent fetal jeopardy. A nonreactive NST or an abnormal modified BPP generally should be followed by additional testing (either a CST or a full BPP). In many circumstances, a positive CST result generally indicates that delivery is warranted. However, the combination of a nonreactive NST and a positive CST result is associated frequently with serious fetal malformation and justifies ultrasonographic investigation for anomalies whenever possible
   2. A BPP score of 6 is considered equivocal; in the term fetus, this score generally should prompt delivery, whereas in the preterm fetus, it should result in a repeat BPP in 24 hours. In the interim, maternal corticosteroid administration should be considered for pregnancies of less than 34 weeks of gestation. Repeat equivocal scores should result either in delivery or continued intensive surveillance. A BPP score of 4 usually indicates that delivery is warranted.

References: See page 140.

Brief Postoperative Cesarean Section Note

Pre-op diagnosis:
   1. 23 year old G_1P_0, estimated gestational age = 40 weeks
   2. Dystocia
   3. Non-reassuring fetal tracing

Post-op diagnosis: Same as above
Procedure: Primary low segment transverse cesarean section
Attending Surgeon, Assistant:
Anesthesia: Epidural
Operative Findings: Weight and sex of infant, APGARs at 1 min and 5 min;

normal uterus, tubes, ovaries.
Cord pH:
Specimens: Placenta, cord blood (type and Rh).
Estimated Blood Loss: 800 cc; no blood replaced.
Fluids, blood and urine output:
Drains: Foley to gravity.
Complications: None
Disposition: Patient sent to recovery room in stable condition.

Cesarean Section Operative Report

Preoperative Diagnosis:
    1. 23 year old G_1P_0, estimated gestational age = 40 weeks
    2. Dystocia
    3. Non-reassuring fetal tracing
Postoperative Diagnosis: Same as above
Title of Operation: Primary low segment transverse cesarean section
Surgeon:
Assistant:
Anesthesia: Epidural
Findings At Surgery: Male infant in occiput posterior presentation. Thin meconium with none below the cords, pediatrics present at delivery, APGAR's 6/8, weight 3980 g. Normal uterus, tubes, and ovaries.
Description of Operative Procedure:
After assuring informed consent, the patient was taken to the operating room and spinal anesthesia was initiated. The patient was placed in the dorsal, supine position with left lateral tilt. The abdomen was prepped and draped in sterile fashion.

A Pfannenstiel skin incision was made with a scalpel and carried through to the level of the fascia. The fascial incision was extended bilaterally with Mayo scissors. The fascial incision was then grasped with the Kocher clamps, elevated, and sharply and bluntly dissected superiorly and inferiorly from the rectus muscles.

The rectus muscles were then separated in the midline, and the peritoneum was tented up, and entered sharply with Metzenbaum scissors. The peritoneal incision was extended superiorly and inferiorly with good visualization of the bladder.

A bladder blade was then inserted, and the vesicouterine peritoneum was identified, grasped with the pick-ups, and entered sharply with the Metzenbaum scissors. This incision was then extended laterally, and a bladder flap was created. The bladder was retracted using the bladder blade. The lower uterine segment was incised in a transverse fashion with the scalpel, then extended bilaterally with bandage scissors. The bladder blade was removed, and the infants head was delivered atraumatically. The nose and mouth were suctioned and the cord clamped and cut. The infant was handed off to the pediatrician. Cord gases and cord blood were sent.

The placenta was then removed manually, and the uterus was exteriorized, and cleared of all clots and debris. The uterine incision was repaired with 1-O chromic in a running locking fashion. A second layer of 1-O chromic was used to obtain excellent hemostasis. The bladder flap was repaired with a 3-O Vicryl in a running fashion. The cul-de-sac was cleared of clots and the uterus was returned to the abdomen. The peritoneum was closed with 3-0 Vicryl. The fascia was reapproximated with O Vicryl in a running fashion. The skin was closed with staples.

The patient tolerated the procedure well. Needle and sponge counts were correct times two. Two grams of Ancef was given at cord clamp, and a sterile dressing was placed over the incision.
Estimated Blood Loss (EBL): 800 cc; no blood replaced (normal blood loss is 500-1000 cc).
Specimens: Placenta, cord pH, cord blood specimens.

Drains: Foley to gravity.
Fluids: Input - 2000 cc LR; Output - 300 cc clear urine.
Complications: None.
Disposition: The patient was taken to the recovery room then postpartum ward in stable condition.

Postoperative Management after Cesarean Section

I. **Post Cesarean Section Orders**
  A. **Transfer:** to post partum ward when stable.
  B. **Vital signs:** q4h x 24 hours, I and O.
  C. **Activity:** Bed rest x 6-8 hours, then ambulate; if given spinal, keep patient flat on back x 8h. Incentive spirometer q1h while awake.
  D. **Diet:** NPO x 8h, then sips of water. Advance to clear liquids, then to regular diet as tolerated.
  E. **IV Fluids:** IV D5 LR or D5 ½ NS at 125 cc/h. Foley to gravity; discontinue after 12 hours. I and O catheterize prn.
  F. **Medications**
    1. Cefazolin (Ancef) 1 gm IVPB x one dose at time of cesarean section.
    2. Nalbuphine (Nubain) 5 to 10 mg SC or IV q2-3h **OR**
    3. Meperidine (Demerol) 50-75 mg IM q3-4h prn pain.
    4. Hydroxyzine (Vistaril) 25-50 mg IM q3-4h prn nausea.
    5. Prochlorperazine (Compazine) 10 mg IV q4-6h prn nausea **OR**
    6. Promethazine (Phenergan) 25-50 mg IV q3-4h prn nausea
  G. **Labs:** CBC in AM.
II. **Postoperative Day #1**
  A. Assess pain, lungs, cardiac status, fundal height, lochia, passing of flatus, bowel movement, distension, tenderness, bowel sounds, incision.
  B. Discontinue IV when taking adequate PO fluids.
  C. Discontinue Foley, and I and O catheterize prn.
  D. Ambulate tid with assistance; incentive spirometer q1h while awake.
  E. Check hematocrit, hemoglobin, Rh, and rubella status.
  F. **Medications**
    1. Acetaminophen/codeine (Tylenol #3) 1-2 PO q4-6h prn pain **OR**
    2. Oxycodone/acetaminophen (Percocet) 1 tab q6h prn pain.
    3. FeSO4 325 mg PO bid-tid.
    4. Multivitamin PO qd, Colace 100 mg PO bid. Mylicon 80 mg PO qid prn bloating.
III. **Postoperative Day #2**
  A. If passing gas and/or bowel movement, advance to regular diet.
  B. Laxatives: Dulcolax supp prn or Milk of magnesia 30 cc PO tid prn. Mylicon 80 mg PO qid prn bloating.
IV. **Postoperative Day #3**
  A. If transverse incision, remove staples and place steri-strips on day 3. If a vertical incision, remove staples on post op day 5.
  B. Discharge home on appropriate medications; follow up in 2 and 6 weeks.

Laparoscopic Bilateral Tubal Ligation Operative Report

Preoperative Diagnosis: Multiparous female desiring permanent sterilization.
Postoperative Diagnosis: Same as above
Title of Operation: Laparoscopic bilateral tubal ligation with Falope rings
Surgeon:
Assistant:

Anesthesia: General endotracheal
Findings At Surgery: Normal uterus, tubes, and ovaries.
Description of Operative Procedure

After informed consent, the patient was taken to the operating room where general anesthesia was administered. The patient was examined under anesthesia and found to have a normal uterus with normal adnexa. She was placed in the dorsal lithotomy position and prepped and draped in sterile fashion. A bivalve speculum was placed in the vagina, and the anterior lip of the cervix was grasped with a single toothed tenaculum. A uterine manipulator was placed into the endocervical canal and articulated with the tenaculum. The speculum was removed from the vagina.

An infraumbilical incision was made with a scalpel, then while tenting up on the abdomen, a Verres needle was admitted into the intraabdominal cavity. A saline drop test was performed and noted to be within normal limits. Pneumoperitoneum was attained with 4 liters of carbon dioxide. The Verres needle was removed, and a 10 mm trocar and sleeve were advanced into the intraabdominal cavity while tenting up on the abdomen. The laparoscope was inserted and proper location was confirmed. A second incision was made 2 cm above the symphysis pubis, and a 5 mm trocar and sleeve were inserted into the abdomen under laparoscopic visualization without complication.

A survey revealed normal pelvic and abdominal anatomy. A Falope ring applicator was advanced through the second trocar sleeve, and the left Fallopian tube was identified, followed out to the fimbriated end, and grasped 4 cm from the cornual region. The Falope ring was applied to a knuckle of tube and good blanching was noted at the site of application. No bleeding was observed from the mesosalpinx. The Falope ring applicator was reloaded, and a Falope ring was applied in a similar fashion to the opposite tube. Carbon dioxide was allowed to escape from the abdomen.

The instruments were removed, and the skin incisions were closed with #3-O Vicryl in a subcuticular fashion. The instruments were removed from the vagina, and excellent hemostasis was noted. The patient tolerated the procedure well, and sponge, lap and needle counts were correct times two. The patient was taken to the recovery room in stable condition.
Estimated Blood Loss (EBL): <10 cc
Specimens: None
Drains: Foley to gravity
Fluids: 1500 cc LR
Complications: None
Disposition: The patient was taken to the recovery room in stable condition.

Postpartum Tubal Ligation Operative Report

Preoperative Diagnosis: Multiparous female after vaginal delivery, desiring permanent sterilization.
Postoperative Diagnosis: Same as above
Title of Operation: Modified Pomeroy bilateral tubal ligation
Surgeon:
Assistant:
Anesthesia: Epidural
Findings At Surgery: Normal fallopian tubes bilaterally
Description of Operative Procedure:

After assuring informed consent, the patient was taken to the operating room and spinal anesthesia administered. A small, transverse, infraumbilical skin incision was made with a scalpel, and the incision was carried down through the underlying fascia until the peritoneum was identified and entered. The left fallopian tube was identified, brought into the incision and grasped with a Babcock clamp. The tube was then followed out to the fimbria. An avascular midsection of the fallopian tube was grasped with a Babcock clamp and brought into a knuckle. The tube was doubly ligated with an O-plain suture and transected. The specimen was sent to pathology. Excellent hemostasis was noted, and the tube was returned to the abdomen. The same procedure was performed on the opposite fallopian tube.

The fascia was then closed with O-Vicryl in a single layer. The skin was closed with 3-O Vicryl in a subcuticular fashion. The patient tolerated the procedure well. Needle and sponge counts were correct times 2.

Estimated Blood Loss (EBL): <20 cc
Specimens: Segments of right and left tubes
Drains: Foley to gravity
Fluids: Input - 500 cc LR; output - 300 cc clear urine
Complications: None
Disposition: The patient was taken to the recovery room in stable condition.
References: See page 140.

Prevention of D Isoimmunization

The morbidity and mortality of Rh hemolytic disease can be significantly reduced by identification of women at risk for isoimmunization and by administration of D immunoglobulin. Administration of D immunoglobulin [RhoGAM, Rho(D) immunoglobulin, RhIg] is very effective in the preventing isoimmunization to the D antigen.

I. **Prenatal testing**
   A. Routine prenatal laboratory evaluation includes ABO and D blood type determination and antibody screen.
   B. At 28-29 weeks of gestation woman who are D negative but not D isoimmunized should be retested for D antibody. If the test reveals that no D antibody is present, prophylactic D immunoglobulin [RhoGAM, Rho(D) immunoglobulin, RhIg] is indicated.
   C. If D antibody is present, D immunoglobulin will not be beneficial, and specialized management of the D isoimmunized pregnancy is undertaken to manage hemolytic disease of the fetus and hydrops fetalis.

II. **Routine administration of D immunoglobulin**
   A. **Abortion.** D sensitization may be caused by abortion. D sensitization occurs more frequently after induced abortion than after spontaneous abortion, and it occurs more frequently after late abortion than after early abortion. D sensitization occurs following induced abortion in 4-5% of susceptible women. All unsensitized, D-negative women who have an induced or spontaneous abortion should be treated with D immunoglobulin unless the father is known to be D negative.
   B. **Dosage** of D immunoglobulin is determined by the stage of gestation. If the abortion occurs before 13 weeks of gestation, 50 mcg of D immunoglobulin prevents sensitization. For abortions occurring at 13 weeks of gestation and later, 300-mcg is given.
   C. **Ectopic pregnancy** can cause D sensitization. All unsensitized, D-negative women who have an ectopic pregnancy should be given D immunoglobulin. The dosage is determined by the gestational age, as described above for abortion.
   D. **Amniocentesis**
      1. D isoimmunization can occur after amniocentesis. D immunoglobulin, 300 mcg, should be administered to unsensitized, D-negative, susceptible patients following first- and second-trimester amniocentesis.
      2. Following third-trimester amniocentesis, 300 mcg of D immunoglobulin should be administered. If amniocentesis is performed and delivery is planned within 48 hours, D immunoglobulin can be withheld until after delivery, when the newborn can be tested for D positivity. If the amniocentesis is expected to precede delivery by more than 48 hours, the patient should receive 300 mcg of D immunoglobulin at the time of amniocentesis.

E. Antepartum prophylaxis
   1. Isoimmunized occurs in 1-2% of D-negative women during the antepartum period. D immunoglobulin, administered both during pregnancy and postpartum, can reduce the incidence of D isoimmunization to 0.3%.
   2. Antepartum prophylaxis is given at 28-29 weeks of gestation. Antibody-negative, Rh-negative gravidas should have a repeat assessment at 28 weeks. D immunoglobulin (RhoGAM, RhIg), 300 mcg, is given to D-negative women. However, if the father of the fetus is known with certainty to be D negative, antepartum prophylaxis is not necessary.

F. Postpartum D immunoglobulin
   1. D immunoglobulin is given to the D negative mother as soon after delivery as cord blood findings indicate that the baby is Rh positive.
   2. A woman at risk who is inadvertently not given D immunoglobulin within 72 hours after delivery should still receive prophylaxis at any time up until two weeks after delivery. If prophylaxis is delayed, it may not be effective.
   3. A quantitative Kleihauer-Betke analysis should be performed in situations in which significant maternal bleeding may have occurred (eg, after maternal abdominal trauma, abruptio placentae, external cephalic version). If the quantitative determination is thought to be more than 30 mL, D immune globulin should be given to the mother in multiples of one vial (300 mcg) for each 30 mL of estimated fetal whole blood in her circulation, unless the father of the baby is known to be D negative.

G. Abruptio placentae, placenta previa, cesarean delivery, intrauterine manipulation, or manual removal of the placenta may cause more than 30 mL of fetal-to-maternal bleeding. In these conditions, testing for excessive bleeding (Kleihauer-Betke test) or inadequate D immunoglobulin dosage (indirect Coombs test) is necessary.

References: See page 140.

Complications of Pregnancy

Nausea, Vomiting and Hyperemesis Gravidarum

At least three-fourths of all pregnant women experience some degree of nausea or vomiting. The clinical presentation may range from mild and self-limited discomfort to pernicious vomiting with dehydration, electrolyte disturbances, and prostration. Illness of this severity is called hyperemesis gravidarum.

I. **Evaluation**
   A. Gestational trophoblastic disease and several other conditions associated with pregnancy predispose women to excessive nausea and vomiting. An appropriate workup for these conditions may include:
      1. History and physical examination
      2. Complete blood count
      3. Urinalysis or urine culture, or both
      4. Serology for hepatitis A, B, and C
      5. Hepatic transaminases
      6. Ultrasound examination of the uterus

Conditions That May Predispose to Excessive Nausea and Vomiting

Viral gastroenteritis
Gestational trophoblastic disease
Hepatitis
Urinary tract infection
Multifetal gestation
Gallbladder disease
Migraine

   B. An assessment of hydration should be completed, and helpful laboratory studies include the following:
      1. Urine-specific gravity
      2. Urine acetone or ketones
      3. Serum acetone
      4. Serum electrolytes
   C. The appearance of acetone in the urine is nonspecific and may follow an overnight fast by a normal gravida. Large amounts of urine acetone or the presence of significant acetone in serum, however, suggest that the pregnant woman is obtaining much of her caloric requirement from lipolysis. This finding, in turn, suggests that she has exhausted glucose and glycogen stores and may benefit from IV therapy

II. **Therapy**
   A. Instruct pregnant patients to eat frequent small meals and to avoid foods that do not appeal to them. The patient should eat small amounts of food that she is able to tolerate.
   B. In early pregnancy, prenatal vitamin and iron pills often are associated with nausea and vomiting and should be avoided if such symptoms occur, although adequate folic acid intake (0.4 mg/day) needs to be assured.
   C. Patients with hyperemesis gravidarum may require hospitalization and IV hydration. The average woman with no severe electrolyte abnormalities should be given IV therapy with 0.5 normal saline in 5% dextrose with 20 mEq KCL in each liter to run continuously at 125 mL/hr. Women with persistent vomiting may develop hypokalemia and hypochloremic alkalosis. In such instances, additional potassium chloride may be required. The concentration of potassium chloride

should not exceed 30 mEq/L. In rare instances, prolonged nausea and vomiting may require total parenteral nutrition.

    D. Medications. The medications used include agents with antihistamine or phenothiazine characteristics, or both. Common drug regimens are:

        1. Promethazine (Phenergan), 12.5 to 25.0 mg every 6 hours po or rectally

        2. Hydroxyzine (Vistaril), 25 to 50 mg every 6 hours po or rectally

        3. Trimethobenzamide (Tigan), 200 mg every 6 hours po

        4. Prochlorperazine (Compazine), 5 to 10 mg orally every 6 hr or 10 mg IM every 4 hours, or 25 mg suppository per rectum twice a day.

References: See page 140.

Spontaneous Abortion

Abortion is defined as termination of pregnancy resulting in expulsion of an immature, nonviable fetus. A fetus of <20 weeks gestation or a fetus weighing <500 gm is considered an abortus. Spontaneous abortion occurs in 15% of all pregnancies.

I. Threatened abortion is defined as vaginal bleeding occurring in the first 20 weeks of pregnancy, without the passage of tissue or rupture of membranes.

    A. Symptoms of pregnancy (nausea, vomiting, fatigue, breast tenderness, urinary frequency) are usually present.

    B. Speculum exam reveals blood coming from the cervical os without amniotic fluid or tissue in the endocervical canal.

    C. The internal cervical os is closed, and the uterus is soft and enlarged appropriate for gestational age.

    D. Differential diagnosis

        1. Benign and malignant lesions. The cervix often bleeds from an ectropion of friable tissue. Hemostasis can be accomplished by applying pressure for several minutes with a large swab or by cautery with a silver nitrate stick. Atypical cervical lesions are evaluated with colposcopy and biopsy.

        2. Disorders of pregnancy

            a. Hydatidiform mole may present with early pregnancy bleeding, passage of grape-like vesicles, and a uterus that is enlarged in excess of that expected from dates. An absence of heart tones by Doppler after 12 weeks is characteristic. Hyperemesis, preeclampsia, or hyperthyroidism may be present. Ultrasonography confirms the diagnosis.

            b. Ectopic pregnancy should be excluded when first trimester bleeding is associated with pelvic pain. Orthostatic light-headedness, syncope or shoulder pain (from diaphragmatic irritation) may occur.

                (1) Abdominal tenderness is noted, and pelvic examination reveals cervical motion tenderness.

                (2) Serum beta-HCG is positive.

    E. Laboratory tests

        1. Complete blood count. The CBC will not reflect acute blood loss.

        2. Quantitative serum beta-HCG level may be positive in nonviable gestations since beta-HCG may persist in the serum for several weeks after fetal death.

        3. Ultrasonography should detect fetal heart motion by 7 weeks gestation or older. Failure to detect fetal heart motion after 9 weeks gestation should prompt consideration of curettage.

    F. Treatment of threatened abortion

        1. Bed rest with sedation and abstinence from intercourse.

        2. The patient should report increased bleeding (>normal menses), cramping, passage of tissue, or fever. Passed tissue should be saved for examination.

II. Inevitable abortion is defined as a threatened abortion with a dilated cervical os. Menstrual-like cramps usually occur.

A. Differential diagnosis

1. **Incomplete abortion** is diagnosed when tissue has passed. Tissue may be visible in the vagina or endocervical canal.
2. **Threatened abortion** is diagnosed when the internal os is closed and will not admit a fingertip.
3. **Incompetent cervix** is characterized by dilatation of the cervix without cramps.

B. Treatment of inevitable abortion

1. Surgical evacuation of the uterus is necessary.
2. D immunoglobulin (RhoGAM) is administered to Rh-negative, unsensitized patients to prevent isoimmunization. Before 13 weeks gestation, the dosage is 50 mcg IM; at 13 weeks gestation, the dosage is 300 mcg IM.

III. **Incomplete abortion** is characterized by cramping, bleeding, passage of tissue, and a dilated internal os with tissue present in the vagina or endocervical canal. Profuse bleeding, orthostatic dizziness, syncope, and postural pulse and blood pressure changes may occur.

A. Laboratory evaluation

1. **Complete blood count.** CBC will not reflect acute blood loss.
2. **Rh typing**
3. **Blood typing and cress-matching.**
4. **Karyotyping** of products of conception is completed if loss is recurrent.

B. Treatment

1. **Stabilization.** If the patient has signs and symptoms of heavy bleeding, at least 2 large-bore IV catheters (<16 gauge) are placed. Lactate Ringer's or normal saline with 40 U oxytocin/L is given IV at 200 mL/hour or greater.
2. Products of conception are removed from the endocervical canal and uterus with a ring forceps. Immediate removal decreases bleeding. Curettage is performed after vital signs have stabilized.
3. **Suction dilation and curettage**
   a. Analgesia consists of meperidine (Demerol), 35-50 mg IV over 3-5 minutes until the patient is drowsy.
   b. The patient is placed in the dorsal lithotomy position in stirrups, prepared, draped, and sedated.
   c. A weighted speculum is placed intravaginally, the vagina and cervix are cleansed, and a paracervical block is placed.
   d. Bimanual examination confirms uterine position and size, and uterine sounding confirms the direction of the endocervical canal.
   e. Mechanical dilatation is completed with dilators if necessary. Curettage is performed with an 8 mm suction curette, with a single-tooth tenaculum on the anterior lip of the cervix.
4. **Post-curettage.** After curettage, a blood count is ordered. If the vital signs are stable for several hours, the patient is discharged with instructions to avoid coitus, douching, or the use of tampons for 2 weeks. Ferrous sulfate and ibuprofen are prescribed for pain.
5. **Rh-negative,** unsensitized patients are given IM RhoGAM.
6. **Methylergonovine (Methergine),** 0.2 mg PO q4h for 6 doses, is given if there is continued moderate bleeding.

IV. **Complete abortion**

A. A complete abortion is diagnosed when complete passage of products of conception has occurred. The uterus is well contracted, and the cervical os may be closed.

B. Differential diagnosis

1. Incomplete abortion
2. **Ectopic pregnancy.** Products of conception should be examined grossly and submitted for pathologic examination. If no fetal tissue or villi are observed grossly, ectopic pregnancy must be excluded by ultrasound.

C. Management of complete abortion

1. Between 8 and 14 weeks, curettage is necessary because of the high

probability that the abortion was incomplete.
2. D immunoglobulin (RhoGAM) is administered to Rh-negative, unsensitized patients.
3. Beta-HCG levels are obtained weekly until zero. Incomplete abortion is suspected if beta-HCG levels plateau or fail to reach zero within 4 weeks.

V. Missed abortion is diagnosed when products of conception are retained after the fetus has expired. If products are retained, a severe coagulopathy with bleeding often occurs.
   A. Missed abortion should be suspected when the pregnant uterus fails to grow as expected or when fetal heart tones disappear.
   B. Amenorrhea may persist, or intermittent vaginal bleeding, spotting, or brown discharge may be noted.
   C. **Ultrasonography** confirms the diagnosis.
   D. **Management of missed abortion**
      1. CBC with platelet count, fibrinogen level, partial thromboplastin time, and ABO blood typing and antibody screen are obtained.
      2. **Evacuation** of the uterus is completed after fetal death has been confirmed. Dilation and evacuation by suction curettage is appropriate when the uterus is less than 12-14 weeks gestational size.
      3. D immunoglobulin (RhoGAM) is administered to Rh-negative, unsensitized patients.

References: See page 140.

Antepartum Urinary Tract Infection

Four to 8% of pregnant women will develop asymptomatic bacteriuria, and 1-3% will develop symptomatic cystitis with dysuria. Pyelonephritis develops in 25-30% of women with untreated bacteriuria.

I. **Asymptomatic bacteriuria** is diagnosed by prenatal urine culture screening, and it is defined as a colony count $\geq 10^5$ organisms per milliliter. Patients with symptomatic cystitis should be treated with oral antibiotics without waiting for urine culture results.
   A. Approximately 80% of infections are caused by Escherichia coli; 10-15% are due to Klebsiella pneumonia or Proteus species; 5% or less are caused by group B streptococci, enterococci, or staphylococci.
   B. **Antibiotic therapy**
      1. Cystitis or asymptomatic bacteriuria is treated for 3 days. A repeat culture is completed after therapy.
      2. Nitrofurantoin monohydrate (Macrobid) 100 mg PO bid **OR**
      3. Nitrofurantoin (Macrodantin) 100 mg PO qid **OR**
      4. Amoxicillin 250-500 mg PO tid **OR**
      5. Cephalexin (Keflex) 250-500 mg PO qid.

II. **Pyelonephritis**
   A. In pregnancy, pyelonephritis can progress rapidly to septic shock and may cause preterm labor. Upper tract urinary infections are associated with an increased incidence of fetal prematurity. Pyelonephritis is characterized by fever, chills, nausea, uterine contractions, and dysuria.
   B. Physical exam usually reveals fever and costovertebral angle tenderness.
   C. The most common pathogens are Escherichia coli and Klebsiella pneumoniae.
   D. Patients should be hospitalized for intravenous antibiotics and fluids. Pyelonephritis is treated with an intravenous antibiotic regimen to which the infectious organism is sensitive for 7-10 days.
   E. Cefazolin (Ancef) 1-2 gm IVPB q8h **OR**
   F. Ampicillin 1 gm IVPB q4-6h **AND**
   G. Gentamicin 2 mg/kg IVPB then 1.5 mg/kg IV q8h **OR**
   H. Ampicillin/sulbactam (Unasyn) 1.5-3 gm IVPB q6h.
   I. Bedrest in the semi Fowler's position on the side opposite affected kidney may help to relieve the pain. Patients with continued fever and pain for

more than 48 to 72 hours may have a resistant organism, obstruction, perinephric abscess, or an infected calculus or cyst.
- **J. Oral antibiotics** are initiated once fever and pain have resolved for at least 24 hours.
  1. **Nitrofurantoin monohydrate (Macrobid)** 100 mg PO bid x 7-10 days, then 100 mg PO qhs **OR**
  2. **Nitrofurantoin (Macrodantin)** 100 mg PO qid x 7-10 days, then 100 mg PO qhs **OR**
  3. **Cephalexin (Keflex)** 500 mg PO qid x 7-10 days **OR**
  4. **Amoxicillin**, 250 mg tid; sulfisoxazole, 500 mg qid x 7-10 days
  5. **Contraindicated Antibiotics.** Sulfonamides should not be used within four weeks of delivery because kernicterus is a theoretical risk. Aminoglycosides should be used for only short periods because of fetal ototoxicity and nephrotoxicity.
  6. Nitrofurantoin and sulfonamides may cause hemolysis in patients with glucose 6-phosphate dehydrogenase deficiency.
  7. After successful therapy, cultures are rechecked monthly during pregnancy, and subsequent infections are treated. Antibiotic prophylaxis is recommended for women with two or more bladder infections or one episode of pyelonephritis during pregnancy. Reinfection is treated for 10 days, then low dose prophylaxis is initiated until 2 weeks postpartum. Prophylactic therapy includes nitrofurantoin (Macrodantin), 100 mg at bedtime or sulfisoxazole (Gantrisin) 0.5 gm bid.

References: See page 140.

Trauma During Pregnancy

Trauma is the leading cause of nonobstetric death in women of reproductive age. Six percent of all pregnancies are complicated by some type of trauma.

- **I. Mechanism of injury**
  - **A. Blunt abdominal trauma**
    1. Blunt abdominal trauma secondary to motor vehicle accidents is the leading cause of nonobstetric-related fetal death during pregnancy, followed by falls and assaults. Uterine rupture or laceration, retroperitoneal hemorrhage, renal injury and upper abdominal injuries may also occur after blunt trauma.
    2. **Abruptio placentae** occurs in 40-50% of patients with major traumatic injuries and in up to 5% of patients with minor injuries.
    3. **Clinical findings in blunt abdominal trauma.** Vaginal bleeding, uterine tenderness, uterine contractions, fetal tachycardia, late decelerations, fetal acidosis, and fetal death.
    4. **Detection of abruptio placentae.** Beyond 20 weeks of gestation, external electronic monitoring can detect uterine contractile activity. The presence of vaginal bleeding and tetanic or hypertonic contractions is presumptive evidence of abruptio placentae.
    5. **Uterine rupture**
       a. Uterine rupture is an infrequent but life-threatening complication. It usually occurs after a direct abdominal impact.
       b. Findings of uterine rupture range from subtle (uterine tenderness, nonreassuring fetal heart rate pattern) to severe, with rapid onset of maternal hypovolemic shock and death.
    6. **Direct fetal injury** is an infrequent complication of blunt trauma.
       a. The fetus is more frequently injured as a result of hypoxia from blood loss or abruption.
       b. In the first trimester the uterus is well protected by the maternal pelvis; therefore, minor trauma usually does not usually cause miscarriage in the first trimester.

    B. **Penetrating trauma**
       1. Penetrating abdominal trauma from gunshot and stab wounds during pregnancy has a poor prognosis.
       2. Perinatal mortality is 41-71%. Maternal mortality is less than 5%.

II. **Major trauma in pregnancy**
    A. **Initial evaluation of major abdominal trauma** in pregnant patients does not differ from evaluation of abdominal trauma in a nonpregnant patient.
    B. **Maintain airway, breathing, and circulatory volume.** Two large-bore (14-16-gauge) intravenous lines are placed.
    C. **Oxygen** should be administered by mask or endotracheal intubation. Maternal oxygen saturation should be kept at >90% (an oxygen partial pressure [pO_2] of 60 mm Hg).
    D. **Volume resuscitation**
       1. Crystalloid in the form of lactated Ringer's or normal saline should be given as a 3:1 replacement for the estimated blood loss over the first 30-60 minutes of acute resuscitation.
       2. O-negative packed red cells are preferred if emergent blood is needed before the patient's own blood type is known.
       3. A urinary catheter should be placed to measure urine output and observe for hematuria.
    E. **Deflection of the uterus** off the inferior vena cava and abdominal aorta can be achieved by placing the patient in the lateral decubitus position. If the patient must remain supine, manual deflection of the uterus to the left and placement of a wedge under the patient's hip or backboard will tilt the patient.
    F. **Secondary survey.** Following stabilization, a more detailed secondary survey of the patient, including fetal evaluation, is performed.

III. **Minor trauma in pregnancy**
    A. **Clinical evaluation**
       1. Pregnant patients who sustain seemingly minimal trauma require an evaluation to exclude significant injuries. Common "minor" trauma include falls, especially in the third trimester, blows to the abdomen, and "fender benders" motor vehicle accidents.
       2. The patient should be questioned about seat belt use, loss of consciousness, pain, vaginal bleeding, rupture of membranes, and fetal movement.
       3. **Physical examination**
         a. Physical examination should focus on upper abdominal tenderness (liver or spleen damage), flank pain (renal trauma), uterine pain (placental abruption, uterine rupture), and pain over the symphysis pubis (pelvic fracture, bladder laceration, fetal skull fracture).
         b. A search for orthopedic injuries should be completed.
    B. **Management of minor trauma**
       1. The minor trauma patient with a fetus that is less than 20 weeks gestation (not yet viable), with no significant injury can be safely discharged after documentation of fetal heart rate. Patients with potentially viable fetuses (over 20 weeks of gestation) require fetal monitoring, laboratory tests and ultrasonographic evaluation.
       2. A complete blood count, urinalysis (hematuria), blood type and screen (to check Rh status), and coagulation panel, including measurement of the INR, PTT, fibrinogen and fibrin split products, should be obtained. The coagulation panel is useful if any suspicion of abruption exists.
       3. **The Kleihauer-Betke (KB) test**
         a. This test detects fetal red blood cells in the maternal circulation. A KB stain should be obtained routinely for any pregnant trauma patient whose fetus is over 12 weeks.
         b. Regardless of the patient's blood type and Rh status, the KB test can help determine if fetomaternal hemorrhage has occurred.
         c. The KB test can also be used to determine the amount of Rho(D) immunoglobulin (RhoGAM) required in patients who are Rh-negative.
         d. A positive KB stain indicates uterine trauma, and any patient with a

positive KB stain should receive at least 24 hours of continuous uterine and fetal monitoring and a coagulation panel.

4. **Ultrasonography** is less sensitive for diagnosing abruption than is the finding of uterine contractions on external tocodynamometry. Absence of sonographic evidence of abruption does not completely exclude an abruption.

5. Patients with abdominal pain, significant bruising, vaginal bleeding, rupture of membranes, or uterine contractions should be admitted to the hospital for overnight observation and continuous fetal monitor.

6. Uterine contractions and vaginal bleeding are suggestive of abruption. Even if vaginal bleeding is absent, the presence of contractions is still a concern, since the uterus can contain up to 2 L of blood from a concealed abruption.

7. Trauma patients with no uterine contraction activity, usually do not have abruption, while patients with greater than one contraction per 10 minutes (6 per hour) have a 20% incidence of abruption.

References: See page 140.

Diabetes and Pregnancy

Pregnancies complicated with gestational diabetes have an increased risk of maternal and perinatal complications, long-term maternal morbidity, and morbidity to the offspring. The causes of perinatal morbidity are neonatal hypoglycemia, hyperbilirubinemia, hypocalcemia, polycythemia, macrosomia birth weight more than 9 lbs (or 4 kg), and with that the problem shoulder dystocia, an abnormal apgar score, and Erb's palsy.

Risk Factors for Gestational Diabetes
• Maternal age older than 30 years
• Pregravid weight more than 90 kg
• Family history of diabetes
• Race
• Multiparity
• Macrosomia

I. **Diagnosis of gestational diabetes**
   A. The diagnosis of gestational diabetes is usually accomplished early in the third trimester of pregnancy. The one-hour glucola test is the screening test for gestational diabetes. Nonfasting women are given 50 grams of glucose in a flavored solution, and their blood is taken one hour after ingestion. If the blood sugar equals or exceeds 140 mg/dL, then women are asked to take a three-hour glucose tolerance test (GTT).
   B. For the three-hour GTT, women are advised to consume an unrestricted diet containing at least 150 grams of carbohydrates daily three days prior to testing. They are asked to fast for 10-14 hours prior to testing. All tests are performed in the morning. Blood is drawn fasting and at 1, 2, and 3 hours postingestion of a 100-gram glucose-containing solution. If any two (out of 4) or more results are abnormal, then they are diagnosed as having gestational diabetes.

Criteria for Gestational Diabetes	
Fasting	105 mg/dL
1 hour	190 mg/dL

2 hour	165 mg/dL
3 hour	145 mg/dL

Any two or more abnormal results are diagnostic of gestational diabetes.

II. Management

A. **Dietary management.** The meal schedule should consist of three meals a day with one or two snacks interspersed as well as a snack after dinner. Initial diet should consist of an intake of 35 kcal/kg of ideal body weight for most nonunderweight, nonobese patients. Generally a diet consisting of complex carbohydrates (as opposed to simple sugars), soluble fiber, low in fat, while reduced in saturated fats, is recommended.

B. **Exercise management** Participation in aerobic activities three to four days per week for 15-30 minutes per session may be beneficial. Pulse should not exceed 70-80% of her maximal heart rate adjusted for her age (target heart rate = [220 - age] x 70%). This will be between 130-150 bpm.

C. **Insulin.** The criteria for insulin therapy are failure of dietary and exercise management. If the fasting blood sugar is greater than 95, if the one-hour postprandial blood sugar is equal to or greater than 140, or if the two-hour postprandial blood sugar is equal to or greater than 120, then the patient needs tighter control of the blood sugar. Human insulin is the drug of choice for treatment of gestational or pregestational diabetes. Insulin dosing of 0.7-1.0 U/kg, depending on the patient's week of gestation (longer gestation usually requiring the higher dose), is recommended. The patient may require a combination of long-acting NPH with regular insulin.

Give 2/3 of total daily requirement in the AM; divide AM dose into 2/3 NPH and 1/3 regular. Give 1/3 of daily requirement in evening: ½ as NPH and ½ as regular insulin. Adjust doses by no more than 20% at a time.

D. **Blood glucose monitoring.** In gestational diabetes the blood sugar should be checked at least four times daily. The fasting blood sugar should not exceed 95 mg/dL and the two-hour postprandial blood sugar should not exceed 120 mg/dL.

Treatment Goals for Gestational Diabetes Mellitus

Time	Blood Sugar	Blood Sugar
Fasting	95 mg/dL	< 5.3 mmol/L
1 hr postprandial	140 mg/dL	< 7.8 mmol/L
2 hr postprandial	120 mg/dL	< 6.7 mmol/L

E. **Fetal surveillance**

1. **Kick counts** are a simple, inexpensive way of measuring fetal well-being. Kick counts are usually done after a meal or snack. The patient lies on her left side and counts the number of fetal movements over a one-hour period. When she gets to 10 movements, she has accomplished a reassuring test of fetal well-being.

2. **Ultrasonography** is useful in diagnosing abnormalities in fetal growth (such as macrosomia, intrauterine growth retardation, or polyhydramnios). Scanning the crown rump length in the first trimester can confirm dates. Fetal ultrasonography used in the third trimester can give an estimated fetal weight and allow measurement of the abdominal circumference.

3. **A maternal serum alpha-fetal protein** level is important at 16-18 weeks because of the increased incidence of open neural tube defects

in diabetic pregnancies.

4. **Nonstress testing** is also used after 32 weeks to evaluate fetal well-being of pregestational or gestational diabetic pregnancies. Two accelerations of the heart rate from the baseline over a 20-minute period of monitoring is a favorable response.

5. **Biophysical profiles** combine ultrasonography with nonstress testing. This allows evaluation of amniotic fluid volume as well as abnormalities in fetal growth or development. A score is derived from observing fetal activity, tone, breathing, and amniotic fluid. A score of 8 or above is reassuring.

F. **Labor and delivery**

1. **Delivery** after 38 weeks increases the probability of the infant developing macrosomia. Unless the pregnancy is complicated by macrosomia, polyhydramnios, poor control of diabetes, or other obstetrical indications (such as pre-eclampsia or intrauterine growth retardation), delivery at term is recommended.

2. **Amniocentesis** is usually indicated if delivery is decided on prior to 38 weeks. A lecithin to sphingomyelin (L/S) ratio of 2 or greater along with the presence of phosphatidylglycerol is what is recommended as being indicative of lung maturity for elective delivery before 38 weeks. After 38 weeks, if the patient has good dates and had a first or second trimester ultrasound that confirms the gestational age, an amniocentesis does not need to be performed.

3. **Induction** is recommended if the patient does not spontaneously go into labor between 39 and 40 weeks. At 40 weeks if her cervix is unfavorable, prostaglandin agents may be necessary to ripen the cervix.

4. **Diabetes management during labor** requires good control of blood sugar while avoiding hypoglycemia. Many patients require no insulin during labor. Blood sugar should be checked every 1-2 hours during labor. Dextrose will need to be given intravenously if the patient's blood sugar falls below 70 mg/dL. Short-acting regular insulin may need to be given intravenously for blood sugars rising above 140 mg/dL (7.8 mmol/L). Plasma glucose should be maintained at 100 to 130 mg/dL.

G. **Postpartum care.** Insulin requirements decrease after the placenta has been delivered. If the patient was on an insulin infusion during labor the dose should be cut in half at this time. For patients with pregestational diabetes the pre-pregnancy insulin dose should be reinitiated after the patient is able to eat.

Low-dosage Constant Insulin Infusion for the Intrapartum Period		
Blood Glucose (mg/100 mL)	**Insulin Dosage (U/h)**	**Fluids (125 mL/h)**
<100	0	5%dextrose/Lactated Ringer's solution
100-140	1.0	5% dextrose/Lactated Ringer's solution
141-180	1.5	Normal saline
181-220	2.0	Normal saline
>220	2.5	Normal saline
Dilution is 25 U of regular insulin in 250 mL of normal saline, with 25 mL flushed through line, administered intravenously.		

H. **Elective cesarean delivery**
1. An estimated fetal weight of greater than 4500 g is an indication for cesarean delivery to avoid birth trauma.
2. Elective cesarean delivery is scheduled for early morning. The usual morning insulin dose is withheld, and glucose levels are monitored hourly. A 5% dextrose solution is initiated and an insulin infusion is initiated. After delivery, intravenous dextrose is continued, and glucose levels are checked every 4-6 hours. In the postpartum period, short-acting insulin is administered if the glucose level rises above 200 mg/dL.
3. For patients with pregestational diabetes, once the patient begins a regular diet, subcutaneous insulin can be reinstituted at dosages substantially lower than those given in the third trimester. It is helpful if the pregestational dose is known.

References: See page 140.

Premature Rupture of Membranes

Premature rupture of membranes (PROM) is the most common diagnosis associated with preterm delivery. The incidence of this disorder to be 7-12%. In pregnancies of less than 37 weeks of gestation, preterm birth (and its sequelae) and infection are the major concerns after PROM.

I. **Pathophysiology**
   A. **Premature rupture of membranes** is defined as rupture of membranes prior to the onset of labor.
   B. **Preterm premature rupture of membranes** is defined as rupture of membranes prior to term.
   C. **Prolonged rupture of membranes** consists of rupture of membranes for more than 24 hours.
   D. **The latent period** is the time interval from rupture of membranes to the onset of regular contractions or labor.
   E. Many cases of preterm PROM are caused by idiopathic weakening of the membranes, many of which are caused by subclinical infection. Other causes of PROM include hydramnios, incompetent cervix, abruptio placentae, and amniocentesis.
   F. At term, about 8% of patients will present with ruptured membranes prior to the onset of labor.

II. **Maternal and neonatal complications**
   A. Labor usually follows shortly after the occurrence of PROM. Ninety percent of term patients and 50% of preterm patients go into labor within 24 hours after rupture.
   B. Patients who do not go into labor immediately are at increasing risk of infection as the duration of rupture increases. Chorioamnionitis, endometritis, sepsis, and neonatal infections may occur.
   C. Perinatal risks with preterm PROM are primarily complications from immaturity, including respiratory distress syndrome, intraventricular hemorrhage, patent ductus arteriosus, and necrotizing enterocolitis.
   D. Premature gestational age is a more significant cause of neonatal morbidity than is the duration of membrane rupture.

III. **Diagnosis of premature rupture of membranes**
   A. Diagnosis is based on history, physical examination, and laboratory testing. The patient's history alone is correct in 90% of patients. Urinary leakage or excess vaginal discharge is sometimes mistaken for PROM.
   B. **Sterile speculum exam** is the first step in confirming the suspicion of PROM. Digital examination should be avoided because it increases the risk of infection.
      1. The general appearance of the cervix should be assessed visually, and prolapse of the umbilical cord or a fetal extremity should be excluded. Cultures for group B streptococcus, gonorrhea, and chlamydia are obtained.

2. A pool of fluid in the posterior vaginal fornix supports the diagnosis of PROM.
3. The presence of amniotic fluid is confirmed by nitrazine testing for an alkaline pH. Amniotic fluid causes nitrazine paper to turn dark blue because the pH is above 6.0-6.5. Nitrazine may be false-positive with contamination from blood, semen, or vaginitis.
4. If pooling and nitrazine are both non-confirmatory, a swab from the posterior fornix should be smeared on a slide, allowed to dry, and examined under a microscope for "ferning," indicating amniotic fluid.
5. Ultrasound examination for oligohydramnios is useful to confirm the diagnosis, but oligohydramnios may be caused by other disorders besides PROM.

IV. Assessment of premature rupture of membranes
A. The gestational age must be carefully assessed. Menstrual history, prenatal exams, and previous sonograms are reviewed. An ultrasound examination should be performed.
B. The patient should be evaluated for the presence of chorioamnionitis [fever (over 38°C), leukocytosis, maternal and fetal tachycardia, uterine tenderness, foul-smelling vaginal discharge].
C. The patient should be evaluated for labor, and a sterile speculum examination should assess cervical change.
D. The fetus should be evaluated with heart rate monitoring because PROM increases the risk of umbilical cord prolapse and fetal distress caused by oligohydramnios.

V. Management of premature rupture of membranes
A. Term patients
1. At 36 weeks and beyond, management of PROM consists of delivery. Patients in active labor should be allowed to progress.
2. Patients with chorioamnionitis, who are not in labor, should be immediately induced with oxytocin (Pitocin).
3. Patients who are not yet in active labor (in the absence of fetal distress, meconium, or clinical infection) may be discharged for 48 hours, and labor usually follows. If labor has not begun within a reasonable time after rupture of membranes, induction with oxytocin (Pitocin) is appropriate. Use of prostaglandin E2 is safe for cervical ripening.

B. Preterm patients
1. Preterm patients with PROM prior to 36 weeks are managed expectantly. Delivery is delayed for the patients who are not in labor, not infected, and without evidence of fetal distress.
2. Patients should be monitored for infection. Cultures for gonococci, Chlamydia, and group B streptococci are obtained. Symptoms, vital signs, uterine tenderness, odor of the lochia, and leukocyte counts are monitored.
3. Suspected occult chorioamnionitis is diagnosed by amniocentesis for Gram stain and culture, which will reveal gram positive cocci in chains.
4. Ultrasound examination should be performed to detect oligohydramnios.
5. **Antibiotic prophylaxis for group B Streptococcus.** Intrapartum chemoprophylaxis consists of penicillin G, 5 million units, then 2.5 million units IV every 4 hours until delivery. Ampicillin, 2 g initially and then 1 g IV every 4 hours until delivery, is an alternative. Clindamycin or erythromycin may be used for women allergic to penicillin.
6. Prolonged continuous fetal heart rate monitoring in the initial assessment should be followed by frequent fetal evaluation.
7. Premature labor is the most common outcome of preterm PROM. Tocolytic drugs are often used and corticosteroids are recommended to accelerate fetal pulmonary maturity.
8. Expectant management consists of in-hospital observation. Delivery is indicated for chorioamnionitis, irreversible fetal distress, or premature labor. Once gestation reaches 36 weeks, the patient may be managed as any other term patient with PROM. Another option is to evaluate the fetus at less than 36 weeks for pulmonary maturity and expedite

delivery once maturity is documented by testing of amniotic fluid collected by amniocentesis or from the vagina. A positive phosphatidyl-glycerol test indicates fetal lung maturity.

C. Previable or preterm premature rupture of membranes

1. In patients in whom membranes rupture very early in pregnancy (eg, <25 weeks). There is a relatively low likelihood (<25%) that a surviving infant will be delivered, and infants that do survive will deliver very premature and suffer significant morbidity.

2. **Fetal deformation syndrome.** The fetus suffering from prolonged early oligohydramnios may develop pulmonary hypoplasia, facial deformation, limb contractures, and deformity.

3. Termination of pregnancy is advisable if the gestational age is early. If the patient elects to continue the pregnancy, expectant management with pelvic rest at home is reasonable.

D. Chorioamnionitis

1. Chorioamnionitis requires delivery (usually vaginally), regardless of the gestational age.

2. **Antibiotic therapy**

a. Ampicillin 2 gm IV q4-6h **AND**

b. Gentamicin 100 mg (2 mg/kg) IV load, then 100 mg (1.5 mg/kg) IV q8h.

References: See page 140.

Preterm Labor

Preterm labor is the leading cause of perinatal morbidity and mortality in the United States. It usually results in preterm birth, a complication that affects 8 to 10 percent of births.

Risk Factors for Preterm Labor	

Previous preterm delivery
Low socioeconomic status
Non-white race
Maternal age <18 years or >40 years
Preterm premature rupture of the membranes
Multiple gestation
Maternal history of one or more spontaneous second-trimester abortions
Maternal complications
  --Maternal behaviors
  --Smoking--Illicit drug use
  --Alcohol use
  --Lack of prenatal care
 	
Uterine causes
  --Myomata (particularly submucosal or subplacental)
  --Uterine septum
  --Bicornuate uterus
  --Cervical incompetence
  --Exposure to diethylstilbestrol (DES)
	Infectious causes
	  --Chorioamnionitis
	  --Bacterial vaginosis
	  --Asymptomatic bacteriuria
	  --Acute pyelonephritis
	  --Cervical/vaginal colonization
	Fetal causes
	  --Intrauterine fetal death
	  --Intrauterine growth retardation
	  --Congenital anomalies
	Abnormal placentation
	Presence of a retained intrauterine device

I. **Risk factors for preterm labor.** Preterm labor is characterized by cervical effacement and/or dilatation, and increased uterine irritability that occurs before 37 weeks of gestation. Women with a history of previous preterm delivery carry the highest risk of recurrence, estimated to be between 17 and 37 percent.

Preterm Labor, Threatened or Actual

1. Initial assessment to determine whether patient is experiencing preterm labor
   a. Assess for the following:
      i. Uterine activity
      ii. Rupture of membranes
      iii. Vaginal bleeding
      iv. Presentation
      v. Cervical dilation and effacement
      vi. Station
   b. Reassess estimate of gestational age
2. Search for a precipitating factor/cause
3. Consider specific management strategies, which may include the following:
   a. Intravenous tocolytic therapy (decision should be influenced by gestational age, cause of preterm labor and contraindications)
   b. Corticosteroid therapy (eg, betamethasone, in a dosage of 12 mg IM every 24 hours for a total of two doses)
   c. Antibiotic therapy if specific infectious agent is identified or if preterm premature rupture of the membranes

---

II. **Management of preterm labor**
   A. **Tocolysis**
      1. Tocolytic therapy may offer some short-term benefit in the management of preterm labor. A delay in delivery can be used to administer corticosteroids to enhance pulmonary maturity and reduce the severity of fetal respiratory distress syndrome, and to reduce the risk of intraventricular hemorrhage. No study has convincingly demonstrated an improvement in survival or neonatal outcome with the use of tocolytic therapy alone.
      2. Contraindications to tocolysis include nonreassuring fetal heart rate tracing, eclampsia or severe preeclampsia, fetal demise (singleton), chorioamnionitis, fetal maturity and maternal hemodynamic instability.
      3. Tocolytic therapy is indicated for regular uterine contractions and cervical change (effacement or dilatation). Oral terbutaline (Bricanyl) following successful parenteral tocolysis is not associated with prolonged pregnancy or reduced incidence of recurrent preterm labor.

Tocolytic Therapy for the Management of Preterm Labor

Medication	Mechanism of action	Dosage
Magnesium sulfate	Intracellular calcium antagonism	4 to 6 g loading dose; then 2 to 4 g IV every hour
Terbutaline (Bricanyl)	Beta$_2$-adrenergic receptor agonist sympathomimetic; decreases free intracellular calcium ions	0.25 to 0.5 mg SC every three to four hours
Ritodrine (Yutopar)	Same as terbutaline	0.05 to 0.35 mg per minute IV
Nifedipine (Procardia)	Calcium channel blocker	5 to 10 mg SL every 15 to 20 minutes (up to four times), then 10 to 20 mg orally every four to six hours

Medication	Mechanism of action	Dosage
Indometha-cin (Indocin)	Prostaglandin inhibitor	50- to 100-mg rectal suppository, then 25 to 50 mg orally every six hours

---

Potential Complications Associated With the Use of Tocolytic Agents

Magnesium sulfate
- Pulmonary edema
- Profound hypotension
- Profound muscular paralysis
- Maternal tetany
- Cardiac arrest
- Respiratory depression

Beta-adrenergic agents
- Hypokalemia
- Hyperglycemia
- Hypotension
- Pulmonary edema
- Arrhythmias
- Cardiac insufficiency
- Myocardial ischemia
- Maternal death

Indomethacin (Indocin)
- Renal failure
- Hepatitis
- Gastrointestinal bleeding

Nifedipine (Procardia)
- Transient hypotension

B. **Corticosteroid therapy**
1. Dexamethasone and betamethasone are the preferred corticosteroids for antenatal therapy. Corticosteroid therapy for fetal maturation reduces mortality, respiratory distress syndrome and intraventricular hemorrhage in infants between 24 and 34 weeks of gestation.
2. In women with preterm premature rapture of membranes (PPROM), antenatal corticosteroid therapy reduces the risk of respiratory distress syndrome. In women with PPROM at less than 30 to 32 weeks of gestation, in the absence of clinical chorioamnionitis, antenatal corticosteroid use is recommended because of the high risk of intraventricular hemorrhage at this early gestational age.

Recommended Antepartum Corticosteroid Regimens for Fetal Maturation in Preterm Infants

Medication	Dosage
Betamethasone (Celestone)	12 mg IM every 24 hours for two doses
Dexamethasone	6 mg IM every 12 hours for four doses

C. **Antibiotic therapy**. Group B streptococcal disease continues to be a major cause of illness and death among newborn infants and has been associated with preterm labor. A gestational age of less than 37 weeks is one of the major risk factors for group B streptococcal disease; therefore, prophylaxis is recommended

Recommended Regimens for Intrapartum Antimicrobial Prophylaxis for Perinatal Group B Streptococcal Disease	
Regimen	**Dosage**
Recommended	Penicillin G, 5 million U IV, then 2.5 million U IV every four hours until delivery
Alternative	Ampicillin, 2 g IV loading dose, then 1 g IV every four hours until delivery
In patients allergic to penicillin	
Recommended	Clindamycin (Cleocin), 900 mg IV every eight hours until delivery
Alternative	Erythromycin, 500 mg IV every six hours until delivery

    D. Bed rest. Although bed rest is often prescribed for women at high risk for preterm labor and delivery, there are no conclusive studies documenting its benefit. A recent meta-analysis found no benefit to bed rest in the prevention of preterm labor or delivery.

References: See page 140.

Bleeding in the Second Half of Pregnancy

Bleeding in the second half of pregnancy occurs in 4% of all pregnancies. In 50% of cases, vaginal bleeding is secondary to placental abruption or placenta previa.

I. **Clinical evaluation of bleeding second half of pregnancy**
    A. **History** of trauma or pain and the amount and character of the bleeding should be assessed.
    B. **Physical examination**
        1. Vital signs and pulse pressure are measured. Hypotension and tachycardia are signs of serious hypovolemia.
        2. Fetal heart rate pattern and uterine activity are assessed.
        3. Ultrasound examination of the uterus, placenta and fetus should be completed.
        4. Speculum and digital pelvic examination should not be done until placenta previa has been excluded.
    C. **Laboratory Evaluation**
        1. **Hemoglobin** and hematocrit.
        2. **INR, partial thromboplastin time, platelet count, fibrinogen level, and fibrin split products** are checked when placental abruption is suspected or if there has been significant hemorrhage.
        3. **A red-top tube** of blood is used to perform a bedside clot test.
        4. **Blood type** and cross-match.
        5. **Urinalysis** for hematuria and proteinuria.
        6. The **Apt test** is used to distinguish maternal or fetal source of bleeding. (Vaginal blood is mixed with an equal part 0.25% sodium hydroxide. Fetal blood remains red; maternal blood turns brown.)
        7. **Kleihauer-Betke test** of maternal blood is used to quantify fetal to maternal hemorrhage.
II. **Placental abruption (abruptio placentae)** is defined as complete or partial placental separation from the decidua basalis after 20 weeks gestation.

A. Placental abruption occurs in 1 in 100 deliveries.
B. Factors associated with placental abruption
 1. Preeclampsia and hypertensive disorders
 2. History of placental abruption
 3. High multiparity
 4. Increasing maternal age
 5. Trauma
 6. Cigarette smoking
 7. Illicit drug use (especially cocaine)
 8. Excessive alcohol consumption
 9. Preterm premature rupture of the membranes
 10. Rapid uterine decompression after delivery of the first fetus in a twin gestation or rupture of membranes with polyhydramnios
 11. Uterine leiomyomas
C. Diagnosis of placental abruption
 1. Abruption is characterized by vaginal bleeding, abdominal pain, uterine tenderness, and uterine contractions.
   a. Vaginal bleeding is visible in 80%; bleeding is concealed in 20%.
   b. Pain is usually of sudden onset, constant, and localized to the uterus and lower back.
   c. Localized or generalized uterine tenderness and increased uterine tone are found with severe placental abruption.
   d. An increase in uterine size may occur with placental abruption when the bleeding is concealed. Concealed bleeding may be detected by serial measurements of abdominal girth and fundal height.
   e. Amniotic fluid may be bloody.
   f. Fetal monitoring may detect distress.
   g. Placental abruption may cause preterm labor.
 2. **Uterine contractions** by tocodynamometry is the most sensitive indicator of abruption.
 3. **Laboratory findings** include proteinuria and a consumptive coagulopathy, characterized by decreased fibrinogen, prothrombin, factors V and VIII, and platelets. Fibrin split products are elevated.
 4. **Ultrasonography** has a sensitivity in detecting placental abruption of only 15%.
D. Management of placental abruption
 1. **Mild placental abruption**
   a. If maternal stability and reassuring fetal surveillance are assured and the fetus is immature, close expectant observation with fetal monitoring is justified.
   b. Maternal hematologic parameters are monitored and abnormalities corrected.
   c. Tocolysis with magnesium sulfate is initiated if the fetus is immature.
 2. **Moderate to severe placental abruption**
   a. Shock is aggressively managed.
   b. **Coagulopathy**
     (1) Blood is transfused to replace blood loss.
     (2) Clotting factors may be replaced using cryoprecipitate or fresh-frozen plasma. One unit of fresh-frozen plasma increases fibrinogen by 10 mg/dL. Cryoprecipitate contains 250 mg fibrinogen/unit; 4 gm (15-20 U) is an effective dose.
     (3) Platelet transfusion is indicated if the platelet count is less than 50,000/mcL. One unit of platelets raises the platelet count 5000-10,000/mcL; 4 to 6 U is the smallest useful dose.
   c. **Oxygen** should be administered and urine output monitored with a Foley catheter.
   d. Vaginal delivery is expedited in all but the mildest cases once the mother has been stabilized. Amniotomy and oxytocin (Pitocin) augmentation may be used. Cesarean section is indicated for fetal distress, severe abruption, or failed trial of labor.
III. Placenta previa occurs when any part of the placenta implants in the lower uterine segment. It is associated with a risk of serious maternal hemorrhage.

Placenta previa occurs in 1 in 200 pregnancies. Ninety percent of placenta previas diagnosed in the second trimester resolve spontaneously.

A. **Total placenta previa** occurs when the internal cervical os is completely covered by placenta.

B. **Partial placenta previa** occurs when part of the cervical os is covered by placenta.

C. **Marginal placenta previa** occurs when the placental edge is located within 2 cm of the cervical os.

D. **Clinical evaluation**

    1. Placenta previa presents with a sudden onset of painless vaginal bleeding in the second or third trimester. The peak incidence occurs at 34 weeks. The initial bleeding usually resolves spontaneously and then recurs later in pregnancy.

    2. One fourth of patients present with bleeding and uterine contractions.

E. **Ultrasonography** is accurate in diagnosing placenta previa.

F. **Management of placenta previa**

    1. In a pregnancy ≥ 36 weeks with documented fetal lung maturity, the neonate should be immediately delivered by cesarean section.

    2. Low vertical uterine incision is probably safer in patients with an anterior placenta. Incisions through the placenta should be avoided.

    3. If severe hemorrhage jeopardizes the mother or fetus, cesarean section is indicated regardless of gestational age.

    4. Expectant management is appropriate for immature fetuses if bleeding is not excessive, maternal physical activity can be restricted, intercourse and douching can be prohibited, and the hemoglobin can be maintained at ≥ 10 mg/dL.

    5. Rh immunoglobulin is administered to Rh-negative-unsensitized patients.

    6. Delivery is indicated once fetal lung maturity has been documented.

    7. Tocolysis with magnesium sulfate may be used for immature fetuses.

IV. **Cervical bleeding**

A. Cytologic sampling is necessary.

B. Bleeding can be controlled with cauterization or packing.

C. Bacterial and viral cultures are sometimes diagnostic.

V. **Cervical polyps**

A. Bleeding is usually self-limited.

B. Trauma should be avoided.

C. Polypectomy may control bleeding and yield a histologic diagnosis.

VI. **Bloody show** is a frequent benign cause of late third trimester bleeding. It is characterized by blood-tinged mucus associated with cervical change.

References: See page 140.

Pregnancy-Induced Hypertension

Women with hypertension during pregnancy typically present with few or no symptoms. The incidence of hypertension during pregnancy is 6 to 8 percent.

I. **Pathophysiology**

A. **Chronic hypertension** is defined as hypertension before the pregnancy or early in the pregnancy.

B. **Pregnancy-induced hypertension** occurs in about 5 percent of pregnancies. ACOG defines preeclampsia as pregnancy-induced hypertension accompanied by renal involvement and proteinuria. Eclampsia is preeclampsia that progresses to seizures. The HELLP syndrome (hemolysis, elevated liver enzymes, low platelet count) is a subcategory of pregnancy-induced hypertension.

C. Blood pressure normally declines during the first trimester and reaches a nadir at 20 weeks gestation. Usually, blood pressure returns to baseline by term. This decline in blood pressure is not seen in women with pregnancy-induced hypertension. Women with chronic hypertension may be normotensive during pregnancy until term.

II. Risk factors

A. Nulliparous women have an increased risk for preeclampsia. Women who are multiparous with a single partner are at the lowest risk. Daughters and sisters of women with a history of pregnancy-induced hypertension have an increased risk for the condition. Preeclampsia is more common in women with chronic hypertension or chronic renal disease.

B. A history of preeclampsia is a primary risk factor. Other risk factors include diabetes, antiphospholipid antibody syndrome and molar pregnancy.

III. Diagnosis

A. ACOG defines hypertension in pregnancy as a sustained blood pressure of 140 mm Hg systolic or 90 mm Hg diastolic or greater. The onset of signs and symptoms of pregnancy-induced hypertension is usually after 20 weeks gestation

B. The classic triad of preeclampsia consists of hypertension, edema and proteinuria. A single urinalysis positive for proteinuria correlates poorly with the true level of proteinuria. A 24-hour urine collection that shows more than 300 mg protein per 24 hours is significant.

C. Excessive weight gain and edema are almost universally seen in preeclampsia. However, edema is also extremely common in normal pregnancies during the third trimester. Generalized edema is more significant than dependent edema occurring only in the lower extremities. Weight gain of greater than 1 to 2 lb per week may indicate significant fluid retention. An increasing hematocrit, which reflects intravascular dehydration, also often occurs in preeclampsia.

D. Renal function tests are often abnormal in preeclampsia. In normal pregnancies, the uric acid level declines during pregnancy and then returns to baseline by term. A uric acid level of greater than 5.0 mg per dL may indicate preeclampsia. Creatinine levels decrease from a normal of 1.0 to 1.5 mg per dL to 0.8 mg per dL or less throughout normal pregnancy but are increased in preeclampsia. Decreased renal perfusion may be indicated by the presence of creatinine levels at term that are the same as normal prepregnancy levels.

E. As preeclampsia worsens and with the HELLP syndrome, liver function test results may become abnormal and platelet levels may significantly decrease. Abnormal liver function test results and low platelet levels reflect the severity of preeclampsia and the possibility of development of disseminated intravascular coagulation (DIC).

F. **Severe pregnancy-induced hypertension** is indicated by symptoms of headache, blurred vision or abdominal pain in combination with elevated blood pressure.

G. **Clinical evaluation** of pregnancy-induced hypertension should include symptoms of headache, visual disturbances and abdominal pain. The woman's blood pressure should be taken in a sitting position five minutes after she is seated. The physical examination should include evaluation of the heart, lungs and abdomen, and neurologic system. Signs of end-organ effects, weight gain and edema should be sought.

H. **Laboratory evaluation.** The urine should be tested for protein. A complete blood count with platelet count, urinalysis, creatinine level, uric acid, a 24-hour urine collection, creatinine clearance and liver function tests should be completed. A screen for early DIC, including fibrin-split products, prothrombin time and total fibrinogen, should be done.

I. **Fetal well-being** and placental function should be assessed with a BPP or an amniotic fluid index and NST. Severe pregnancy-induced hypertension can result in fetal growth restriction. An ultrasound to assess fetal weight and gestational age should verify adequate fetal growth.

IV. Treatment

A. Delivery of the fetus is the only cure for pregnancy-induced hypertension.

B. **Mild disease**

1. Women with mild elevations in blood pressure and proteinuria but no

evidence of severe signs or symptoms may be safely observed without immediate treatment or delivery. Women with mild preeclampsia at term should be considered candidates for induction of labor. Mild elevations in blood pressure (<170 mmHg systolic or <105 mmHg diastolic) do not require treatment with antihypertensive medications.

2. **Initial evaluation** may take place in the hospital with fetal monitoring, 24-hour urine collection and monitoring for progression of disease. All women managed as outpatients should be instructed to contact the physician if any symptoms of severe pregnancy-induced hypertension appear. Follow-up should include tests for proteinuria, blood pressure assessment, home health care nursing and frequent clinic visits. Bi-weekly NSTs, amniotic fluid index assessments, BPPs and serial ultrasounds to document appropriate fetal growth are needed to ensure fetal well-being.

3. **Nonstress testing.** The nonstress test is performed after 32 to 34 weeks, 2-3 times a week or more.

4. **Ultrasonic assessment.** A baseline study is completed at 18 to 24 weeks. Monitoring of fetal growth and amniotic fluid index is initiated at 30 to 32 weeks.

C. **Moderate to severe disease**

1. Women with any of the signs and symptoms of severe pregnancy-induced hypertension require hospitalization. Induction of labor is usually indicated to facilitate prompt delivery. Women at greater than 34 weeks gestation are delivered immediately.

2. Treatment for women at earlier gestations (28 to 34 weeks) consists of conservative observation or immediate delivery. Monitoring may include daily antenatal testing, initial invasive monitoring for fluid status, seizure prophylaxis with magnesium sulfate and administration of corticosteroids.

Clinical Manifestations of Severe Disease in Women with Pregnancy-Induced Hypertension

Blood pressure greater than 160 to 180 mm Hg systolic or greater than 110 mm Hg diastolic
Proteinuria greater than 5 g per 24 hours (normal: less than 300 mg per 24 hours)
Elevated serum creatinine
Grand mal seizures (eclampsia)
Pulmonary edema
Oliguria less than 500 mL per 24 hours
Microangiopathic hemolysis
Thrombocytopenia
Hepatocellular dysfunction (elevated ALT, AST)
Intrauterine growth restriction or oligohydramnios
Symptoms suggesting significant end-organ involvement (ie, headache, visual disturbances, epigastric or right upper-quadrant pain)

---

3. **Magnesium sulfate** is an effective treatment for prevention of seizures in preeclampsia. An intravenous loading dose of 4 g over 20 minutes is given, followed by a dosage regimen of 2 to 3 g per hour. Serum drug levels and side effects should be carefully monitored.

4. **Hypertension** should be treated when blood pressure increases to higher than 170 mm Hg systolic or 105 mm Hg diastolic. Treatment consists of intravenous hydralazine (Apresoline), 6.25 to 25.0 mg every four to six hours. Recent studies have also used oral labetalol (Normodyne, Trandate), 600 mg PO qid, or oral nifedipine, 20 mg PO q4h. Maintaining the blood pressure between 140 and 150 mm Hg systolic and between 90 and 100 mm Hg diastolic decreases the risk

of placental hypoperfusion.

5. **Betamethasone (Celestone)** is given to women with a pregnancy between 28 and 34 weeks gestation in order to improve fetal lung maturity and neonatal survival.

V. Intrapartum management of hypertension

A. **Intrapartum prevention of seizures. Magnesium sulfate** is administered to all patients with hypertension at term to prevent seizures when delivery is indicated. An intravenous loading bolus of 4 g IV over 20 minutes, followed by continuous infusion of 2 g/h. When symptomatic magnesium overdose is suspected (apnea, obtundation), it can be reversed by the intravenous administration of 10% calcium gluconate, 10 mL IV over 2 minutes. Magnesium prophylaxis must be continued in the immediate post-partum period, as the risk of seizures is highest in the intrapartum stage and during the first 24 hours following delivery.

B. **Intrapartum blood pressure control**
1. When blood pressure exceeds 105 mmHg diastolic or 170 mmHg systolic blood pressure should be lowered with intravenous hydralazine.
2. Hydralazine is given IV as a 5-10-mg bolus as often as every 20 minutes as necessary. The goal of treatment is a systolic of 140-150 mmHg and a diastolic of 90-100 mmHg.
3. Labetalol, 20 mg, given IV as often as every 10 minutes to a maximum dose of 300 mg, is an acceptable alternative. Unresponsive blood pressure can occasionally require sodium nitroprusside, with central hemodynamic monitoring.

C. **Vaginal delivery** is generally preferable to cesarean delivery, even in patients with manifestations of severe disease. Cervical ripening with prostaglandin E_2 gel may be considered; however, a seriously ill patient with an unfavorable cervix should receive a cesarean section.

References: See page 140.

Herpes Simplex Virus Infections in Pregnancy

Two types of herpes simplex virus have been identified, herpes simplex virus type 1 (HSV-1) and herpes simplex virus type 2 (HSV-2). Initial contact with HSV usually occurs early in childhood and usually involves HSV-1. Herpes simplex virus type 1 causes most nongenital herpetic lesions: eg, herpes labialis, gingivostomatitis, and keratoconjunctivitis. The female genital tract can be infected with HSV-1 or HSV-2. Most genital infection is from HSV-2.

I. Incidence

A. Herpes simplex virus infection of the genital tract is one of the most common viral STDs. The greatest incidence of overt HSV-2 infection occurs in women in their late teens and early twenties. However, 30% of the female population in the United States have antibodies to HSV-2.

B. Newborns may become infected in the perinatal period from contact with infected maternal secretions. Most newborns acquire the virus from asymptomatic mothers without identified lesions.

II. Presentation of infection

A. **Primary infection**
1. Initial genital infection due to herpes may be either asymptomatic or associated with severe symptoms. With symptomatic primary infection, lesions may occur on the vulva, vagina, or cervix, or on all three, between 2 and 14 days following exposure to infectious virus. The initial vesicles rupture and subsequently appear as shallow and eroded ulcers. Inguinal lymphadenopathy is common.
2. Systemic symptoms (malaise, myalgia, and fever) may occur with primary herpetic infections. Local symptoms of pain, dysuria, and soreness of the vulva and vagina are common in both primary and recurrent infections. The lesions of primary infection tends to resolve

within 3 weeks without therapy.

B. Nonprimary first episode disease is associated with fewer systemic manifestations, less pain, a briefer duration of viral shedding, and a more rapid resolution of the clinical lesions in the nonprimary infection. These episodes usually are thought to be the result of an initial HSV-2 infection in the presence of partially protective HSV-1 antibodies.

C. Recurrences of genital HSV infection can be symptomatic or subclinical. The ulcers tend to be limited in size, number, and duration. Local symptoms predominate over systemic symptoms, with many patients indicating increased vaginal discharge or pain. Shedding of the virus from the genital tract without symptoms or signs of clinical lesions (subclinical shedding) is episodic.

D. Neonatal herpes. Most neonatal HSV infection is the consequence of delivery of a neonate through an infected birth canal. There are three categories of neonatal disease: localized disease of the skin, eye, and mouth; central nervous system (CNS) disease with or without skin, eye, and mouth disease; or disseminated disease. Most infected neonates have localized skin, eye, and mouth disease, which generally is a mild illness. Localized disease may progress to encephalitis or disseminated disease. Skin, eye, and mouth disease is usually self-limited. CNS disease has a 15% mortality, and there is a 57% mortality with disseminated disease.

III. Transmission

A. Sexual and direct contact. Herpes simplex virus is transmitted via direct contact with an individual who is infected. Genital-to-genital contact or contact of the genital tract with an area that is infected with HSV, such as oral-to-genital contact, can result in transmission.

B. Maternal-fetal transmission. Vertical transmission rates at the time of vaginal delivery based on the type of maternal disease may be summarized as follows: primary HSV result in 50% transmission; nonprimary first-episode HSV result in 33% transmission; and recurrent HSV result in 0-3% transmission.

IV. Laboratory diagnosis

A. The standard and most sensitive test for detecting HSV from clinical specimens is isolation of the virus by cell culture. More sensitive techniques are increasingly available, such as polymerase chain reaction and hybridization methods.

B. Early primary and nonprimary first-episode ulcers yield the virus in 80% of patients, whereas ulcers from recurrent infections are less likely to be culture-positive; only 40% of crusted lesions contain recoverable virus. When testing for HSV, overt lesions that are not in the ulcerated state should be unroofed and the fluid sampled.

V. Medical management

A. Medical management of women with primary HSV infection during pregnancy. Antiviral therapy for primary infection is recommended for women with primary HSV infection during pregnancy to reduce viral shedding and enhance lesion healing. Primary infection during pregnancy constitutes a higher risk for vertical transmission than does recurrent infection. Suppressive therapy for the duration of the pregnancy should be considered to reduce the potential of continued viral shedding and the likelihood of recurrent episodes.

B. Medical management of women with recurrent HSV infection during pregnancy. Acyclovir should be considered after 36 weeks of gestation in women with recurrent genital herpes infection because it results in a significant decrease in clinical recurrences. The likelihood of cesarean deliveries performed for active infection is not reduced significantly by acyclovir.

C. Acyclovir (Zovirax), a class-C medication, has activity against HSV-1 and HSV-2. In the treatment of primary genital herpes infections, oral acyclovir reduces viral shedding, reduces pain, and heals lesions faster when compared with a placebo. Acyclovir has been shown to be safe in pregnancy and has minimal side effects. Oral dosage is 400 mg tid.

D. **Valacyclovir (Valtrex) and famciclovir (Famvir)** are class-B medications. Their increased bio-availability means that they may require less frequent dosing to achieve the same therapeutic benefits as acyclovir. The U.S. Food and Drug Administration has approved both valacyclovir and famciclovir for the treatment of primary genital herpes, the treatment of episodes of recurrent disease, and the daily treatment for suppression of outbreaks of recurrent genital herpes.

E. Valacyclovir therapy, 500 mg once daily, is effective in suppressing recurrent genital herpes. Suppressive famciclovir therapy requires a 250 mg twice daily.

VI. **Cesarean delivery** is indicated for term pregnancies with active genital lesions or symptoms of vulvar pain or burning, which may indicate an impending outbreak.

VII. **Active HSV and preterm premature rupture of membranes.** In pregnancies remote from term, especially in women with recurrent disease, the pregnancy should be continued to gain benefit from time and glucocorticoids. Treatment with an antiviral agent is indicated.

References: See page 140.

Dystocia and Augmentation of Labor

I. Normal labor
A. First stage of labor
1. The first stage of labor consists of the period from the onset of labor until complete cervical dilation (10 cm). This stage is divided into the latent phase and the active phase.
2. **Latent phase**
   a. During the latent phase, uterine contractions are infrequent and irregular and result in only modest discomfort. They result in gradual effacement and dilation of the cervix.
   b. A prolonged latent phase is one that exceeds 20 hours in the nullipara or one that exceeds 14 hours in the multipara.
3. **Active phase**
   a. The active phase of labor occurs when the cervix reaches 3-4 cm of dilatation.
   b. The active phase of labor is characterized by an increased rate of cervical dilation and by descent of the presenting fetal part.
B. Second stage of labor
1. **The second stage of labor** consists of the period from complete cervical dilation (10 cm) until delivery of the infant. This stage is usually brief, averaging 20 minutes for parous women and 50 minutes for nulliparous women.
2. The duration of the second stage of labor is unrelated to perinatal outcome in the absence of a nonreassuring fetal heart rate pattern as long as progress occurs.

II. Abnormal labor
A. **Dystocia** is defined as difficult labor or childbirth resulting from abnormalities of the cervix and uterus, the fetus, the maternal pelvis, or a combination of these factors.
B. **Cephalopelvic disproportion** is a disparity between the size of the maternal pelvis and the fetal head that precludes vaginal delivery. This condition can rarely be diagnosed in advance.
C. **Slower-than-normal (protraction disorders) or complete cessation of progress (arrest disorder)** are disorders that can be diagnosed only after the parturient has entered the active phase of labor.

III. Assessment of labor abnormalities
A. **Labor abnormalities caused by inadequate uterine contractility (powers).** The minimal uterine contractile pattern of women in spontaneous labor consists of 3 to 5 contractions in a 10-minute period.

B. Labor abnormalities caused by fetal characteristics (passenger)

1. Assessment of the fetus consists of estimating fetal weight and position. Estimations of fetal size, even those obtained by ultrasonography, are frequently inaccurate.
2. In the first stage of labor, the diagnosis of dystocia can not be made unless the active phase of labor and adequate uterine contractile forces have been present.
3. Fetal anomalies such as hydrocephaly, encephalocele, and soft tissue tumors may obstruct labor. Fetal imaging should be considered when malpresentation or anomalies are suspected based on vaginal or abdominal examination or when the presenting fetal part is persistently high.

C. Labor abnormalities due to the pelvic passage (passage)

1. Inefficient uterine action should be corrected before attributing dystocia to a pelvic problem.
2. The bony pelvis is very rarely the factor that limits vaginal delivery of a fetus in cephalic presentation. Radiographic pelvimetry is of limited value in managing most cephalic presentations.
3. Clinical pelvimetry can only be useful to qualitatively identify the general architectural features of the pelvis.

IV. Augmentation of labor

A. Uterine hypocontractility should be augmented only after both the maternal pelvis and fetal presentation have been assessed.

B. Contraindications to augmentation include placenta or vasa previa, umbilical cord prolapse, prior classical uterine incision, pelvic structural deformities, and invasive cervical cancer.

C. Oxytocin (Pitocin)

1. The goal of oxytocin administration is to stimulate uterine activity that is sufficient to produce cervical change and fetal descent while avoiding uterine hyperstimulation and fetal compromise.
2. **Minimally effective uterine activity** is 3 contractions per 10 minutes averaging greater than 25 mm Hg above baseline. A maximum of 5 contractions in a 10-minute period with resultant cervical dilatation is considered adequate.
3. **Hyperstimulation** is characterized by more than five contractions in 10 minutes, contractions lasting 2 minutes or more, or contractions of normal duration occurring within 1 minute of each other.
4. Oxytocin is administered when a patient is progressing slowly through the latent phase of labor or has a protraction or an arrest disorder of labor, or when a hypotonic uterine contraction pattern is identified.
5. A pelvic examination should be performed before initiation of oxytocin infusion.
6. Oxytocin is usually diluted 10 units in 1 liter of normal saline IVPB.

Labor Stimulation with Oxytocin (Pitocin)				
Regimen	Starting Dose (mU/min)	Incremental Increase (mU/min)	Dosage Interval (min)	Maximum Dose (mU/min)
Low-Dose	0.5-1	1	30-40	20

7. **Management of oxytocin-induced hyperstimulation**
   a. The most common adverse effect of hyperstimulation is fetal heart rate deceleration associated with uterine hyperstimulation. Stopping or decreasing the dose of oxytocin may correct the abnormal pattern.
   b. Additional measures may include changing the patient to the lateral decubitus position and administering oxygen or more intravenous fluid.

    c. If oxytocin-induced uterine hyperstimulation does not respond to conservative measures, intravenous terbutaline (0.125-0.25 mg) or magnesium sulfate (2-6 g in 10-20% dilution) may be used to stop uterine contractions.

References: See page 140.

Fetal Macrosomia

Excessive birth weight is associated with an increased risk of maternal and neonatal injury. Macrosomia is defined as a fetus with an estimated weight of more than 4,500 grams, regardless of gestational age.

I. **Diagnosis of macrosomia**
   A. Clinical estimates of fetal weight based on Leopold's maneuvers or fundal height measurements are often inaccurate.
   B. Diagnosis of macrosomia requires ultrasound evaluation; however, estimation of fetal weight based on ultrasound is associated with a large margin of error.
   C. Maternal weight, height, previous obstetric history, fundal height, and the presence of gestational diabetes should be evaluated.

II. **Factors influencing fetal weight**
   A. **Gestational age.** Post-term pregnancy is a risk factor for macrosomia. At 42 weeks and beyond, 2.5% of fetuses weigh more than 4,500 g. Ten to twenty percent of macrosomic infants are post-term fetuses.
   B. **Maternal weight.** Heavy women have a greater risk of giving birth to excessively large infants. Fifteen to 35% of women who deliver macrosomic fetuses weigh 90 kg or more.
   C. **Multiparity.** Macrosomic infants are 2-3 times more likely to be born to parous women.
   D. **Macrosomia in a prior infant.** The risk of delivering an infant weighing more than 4,500 g is increased if a prior infant weighed more than 4,000 g.
   E. **Maternal diabetes**
      1. Maternal diabetes increases the risk of fetal macrosomia and shoulder dystocia.
      2. Cesarean delivery is indicated when the estimated fetal weight exceeds 4,500 g.

III. **Morbidity and mortality**
   A. **Abnormalities of labor.** Macrosomic fetuses have a higher incidence of labor abnormalities and instrumental deliveries.
   B. **Maternal morbidity.** Macrosomic fetuses have a two- to threefold increased rate of cesarean delivery.
   C. **Birth injury**
      1. The incidence of birth injuries occurring during delivery of a macrosomic infant is much greater with vaginal than with cesarean birth. The most common injury is brachial plexus palsy, often caused by shoulder dystocia.
      2. The incidence of shoulder dystocia in infants weighing more than 4,500 g is 8-20%. Macrosomic infants also may sustain fractures of the clavicle or humerus.

IV. **Management of delivery**
   A. If the estimated fetal weight is greater than 4500 gm in the nondiabetic or greater than 4000 gm in the diabetic patient, delivery by cesarean section is indicated.
   B. **Management of shoulder dystocia**
      1. If a shoulder dystocia occurs, an assistant should provide suprapubic pressure to dislodge the impacted anterior fetal shoulder from the symphysis. McRobert maneuver (extreme hip flexion) should be done simultaneously.
      2. If the shoulder remains impacted anteriorly, an ample episiotomy should be cut and the posterior arm delivered.

3. In almost all instances, one or both of these procedures will result in successful delivery. The Zavanelli maneuver consists of replacement of the fetal lead into the vaginal canal and delivery by emergency cesarean section.
4. Fundal pressure is not recommended because it often results in further impaction of the shoulder against the symphysis.

References: See page 140.

Shoulder Dystocia

Shoulder dystocia, defined as failure of the shoulders to deliver following the head, is an obstetric emergency. The incidence varies from 0.6% to 1.4% of all vaginal deliveries. Up to 30% of shoulder dystocias can result in brachial plexus injury; many fewer sustain serious asphyxia or death. Most commonly, size discrepancy secondary to fetal macrosomia is associated with difficult shoulder delivery. Causal factors of macrosomia include maternal diabetes, postdates gestation, and obesity. The fetus of the diabetic gravida may also have disproportionately large shoulders and body size compared with the head.

I. **Prediction**
   A. The diagnosis of shoulder dystocia is made after delivery of the head. The "turtle" sign is the retraction of the chin against the perineum or retraction of the head into the birth canal. This sign demonstrates that the shoulder girdle is resisting entry into the pelvic inlet, and possibly impaction of the anterior shoulder.
   B. Macrosomia has the strongest association. ACOG defines macrosomia as an estimated fetal weight (EFW) greater than 4500 g.
   C. Risk factors for macrosomia include maternal birth weight, prior macrosomia, preexisting diabetes, obesity, multiparity, advanced maternal age, and a prior shoulder dystocia. The recurrence rate has been reported to be 13.8%, nearly seven times the primary rate. Shoulder dystocia occurs in 5.1% of obese women. In the antepartum period, risk factors include gestational diabetes, excessive weight gain, short stature, macrosomia, and postterm pregnancy. Intrapartum factors include prolonged second stage of labor, abnormal first stage, arrest disorders, and instrumental (especially midforceps) delivery. Many shoulder dystocias will occur in the absence of any risk factors.

II. **Management**
   A. Shoulder dystocia is a medical and possibly surgical emergency. Two assistants should be called for if not already present, as well as an anesthesiologist and pediatrician. A generous episiotomy should be cut. The following sequence is suggested:
      1. **McRoberts maneuver:** The legs are removed from the lithotomy position and flexed at the hips, with flexion of the knees against the abdomen. Two assistants are required. This maneuver may be performed prophylactically in anticipation of a difficult delivery.
      2. **Suprapubic pressure:** An assistant is requested to apply pressure downward, above the symphysis pubis. This can be done in a lateral direction to help dislodge the anterior shoulder from behind the pubic symphysis. It can also be performed in anticipation of a difficult delivery. Fundal pressure may increase the likelihood of uterine rupture and is contraindicated.
      3. **Rotational maneuvers:** The Woods' corkscrew maneuver consists of placing two fingers against the anterior aspect of the posterior shoulder. Gentle upward rotational pressure is applied so that the posterior shoulder girdle rotates anteriorly, allowing it to be delivered first. The Rubin maneuver is the reverse of Woods's maneuver. Two fingers are placed against the posterior aspect of the posterior (or anterior) shoulder and forward pressure applied. This results in adduction of the shoulders and displacement of the anterior shoulder

from behind the symphysis pubis.

4. **Posterior arm release:** The operator places a hand into the posterior vagina along the infant's back. The posterior arm is identified and followed to the elbow. The elbow is then swept across the chest, keeping the elbow flexed. The fetal forearm or hand is then grasped and the posterior arm delivered, followed by the anterior shoulder. If the fetus still remains undelivered, vaginal delivery should be abandoned and the Zavanelli maneuver performed followed by cesarean delivery.

5. **Zavanelli maneuver:** The fetal head is replaced into the womb. Tocolysis is recommended to produce uterine relaxation. The maneuver consists of rotation of the head to occiput anterior. The head is then flexed and pushed back into the vagina, followed abdominal delivery. Immediate preparations should be made for cesarean delivery.

6. If cephalic replacement fails, an emergency symphysiotomy should be performed. The urethra should be laterally displaced to minimize the risk of lower urinary tract injury.

B. The McRoberts maneuver alone will successfully alleviate the shoulder dystocia in 42% to 79% of cases. For those requiring additional maneuvers, vaginal delivery can be expected in more than 90%. Finally, favorable results have been reported for the Zavanelli maneuver in up to 90%.

References: See page 140.

Postdates Pregnancy

A term gestation is defined as one completed in 38 to 42 weeks. Pregnancy is considered prolonged or postdates when it exceeds 294 days or 42 weeks from the first day of the last menstrual period (LMP). About 10% of those pregnancies are postdates. The incidence of patients reaching the 42nd week is 3-12%.

I. Morbidity and mortality
A. The rate of maternal, fetal, and neonatal complications increases with gestational age. The cesarean delivery rate more than doubles when passing the 42nd week compared with 40 weeks because of cephalopelvic disproportion resulting from larger infants and by fetal intolerance of labor.

B. Neonatal complications from postdates pregnancies include placental insufficiency, birth trauma from macrosomia, meconium aspiration syndrome, and oligohydramnios.

II. Diagnosis
A. The accurate diagnosis of postdates pregnancy can be made only by proper dating. The estimated date of confinement (EDC) is most accurately determined early in pregnancy. An EDC can be calculated by subtracting 3 months from the first day of the last menses and adding 7 days (Naegele's rule). Other clinical parameters that should be consistent with the EDC include maternal perception of fetal movements (quickening) at about 16 to 20 weeks; first auscultation of fetal heart tones with Doppler ultrasound by 12 weeks; uterine size at early examination (first trimester) consistent with dates; and, at 20 weeks, a fundal height 20 cm above the symphysis pubis or at the umbilicus.

Clinical Estimates of Gestational Age	
Parameter	Gestational age (weeks)
Positive urine hCG	5

Parameter	Gestational age (weeks)
Fetal heart tones by Doppler	11 to 12
Quickening Primigravida Multigravida	 20 16
Fundal height at umbilicus	20

B. In patients without reliable clinical data, ultrasound is beneficial. Ultrasonography is most accurate in early gestation. The crown-rump length becomes less accurate after 12 weeks in determining gestational age because the fetus begins to curve.

III. **Management of the postdates pregnancy**

A. A postdates patient with a favorable cervix should receive induction of labor. Only 8.2% of pregnancies at 42 weeks have a ripe cervix (Bishop score >6). Induction at 41 weeks with PGE_2 cervical ripening lowers the cesarean delivery rate.

B. **Cervical ripening with prostaglandin**

1. Prostaglandin E_2 gel is a valuable tool for improving cervical ripeness and for increasing the likelihood of successful induction.

2. Pre- and postapplication fetal monitoring are usually utilized. If the fetus has a nonreassuring heart rate tracing or there is excessive uterine activity, the use of PGE_2 gel is not advisable. The incidence of uterine hyperstimulation with PGE_2 gel, at approximately 5%, is comparable to that seen with oxytocin. Current PGE_2 modalities include the following:

   a. 2 to 3 mg of PGE_2 suspended in a gel placed intravaginally
   b. 0.5 mg of PGE_2 suspended in a gel placed intracervically (Prepidil)
   c. 10 mg of PGE_2 gel in a sustained-release tape (Cervidil)
   d. 25 µg of PGE_1 (one-fourth of tablet) placed intravaginally every 3 to 4 hours (misoprostol)

C. **Stripping of membranes**, starting at 38 weeks and repeated weekly may be an effective method of inducing labor in post-term women with a favorable cervix. Stripping of membranes is performed by placing a finger in the cervical os and circling 3 times in the plane between the fetal head and cervix.

D. **Expectant management with antenatal surveillance**

1. Begin testing near the end of the 41st week of pregnancy. Antepartum testing consists of the nonstress test (NST) combined with the amniotic fluid index (AFI) twice weekly. The false-negative rate is 6.1/1000 (stillbirth within 1 week of a reassuring test) with twice weekly NSTs.

2. The AFI involves measuring the deepest vertical fluid pocket in each uterine quadrant and summing the four together. Less than 5 cm is considered oligohydramnios, 5 to 8 cm borderline, and greater than 8 cm normal.

E. **Fetal movement counting (kick counts)**. Fetal movement has been correlated with fetal health. It consist of having the mother lie on her side and count fetal movements. Perception of 10 distinct movements in a period of up to 2 hours is considered reassuring. After 10 movements have been perceived, the count may be discontinued.

F. **Delivery** is indicated if the amniotic fluid index is less than 5 cm, a nonreactive non-stress test is identified, or if decelerations are identified on the nonstress test.

G. **Intrapartum management**

1. **Meconium staining** is more common in postdates pregnancies. If oligohydramnios is present, amnioinfusion dilutes meconium and decreases the number of infants with meconium below the vocal cords. Instillation of normal saline through an intrauterine pressure catheter may reduce variable decelerations.

2. **Macrosomia** should be suspected in all postdates gestations. Fetal weight should be estimated prior to labor in all postdates pregnancies. Ultrasonographic weight predictions generally fall within 20% of the actual birth weight.
3. **Management of suspected macrosomia.** The pediatrician and anesthesiologist should be notified so that they can prepare for delivery. Cesarean delivery should be considered in patients with an estimated fetal weight greater than 4500 g and a marginal pelvis, or someone with a previous difficult vaginal delivery with a similarly sized or larger infant.
4. Intrapartum asphyxia is also more common in the postdates pregnancy. Therefore, close observation of the fetal heart rate tracing is necessary during labor. Variable decelerations representing cord compression are frequently seen in postdates pregnancies
5. Cord compression can be treated with amnioinfusion, which can reduce variable decelerations. Late decelerations are more direct evidence of fetal hypoxia. If intermittent, late decelerations are managed conservatively with positioning and oxygen. If persistent late decelerations are associated with decreased variability or an elevated baseline fetal heart rate, immediate evaluation or delivery is indicated. This additional evaluation can include observation for fetal heart acceleration following fetal scalp or acoustic stimulation, or a fetal scalp pH.

References: See page 140.

Induction of Labor

Induction of labor consists of stimulation of uterine contractions before the spontaneous onset of labor for the purpose of accomplishing delivery.

I. **Indications and contraindications**
   A. **Common indications for induction of labor**
      1. Pregnancy-induced hypertension
      2. Premature rupture of membranes
      3. Chorioamnionitis
      4. Suspected fetal jeopardy (eg, severe fetal growth restriction, isoimmunization)
      5. Maternal medical problems (eg, diabetes mellitus, renal disease)
      6. Fetal demise
      7. Postterm pregnancy
   B. **Contraindications to labor induction or spontaneous labor**
      1. Placenta previa or vasa previa
      2. Transverse fetal lie
      3. Prolapsed umbilical cord
      4. Prior classical uterine incision
   C. **Obstetric conditions requiring special caution during induction**
      1. Multifetal gestation
      2. Polyhydramnios
      3. Maternal cardiac disease
      4. Abnormal fetal heart rate patterns not requiring emergency delivery
      5. Grand multiparity
      6. Severe hypertension
      7. Breech presentation
      8. Presenting part above the pelvic inlet
   D. A trial of labor with induction is not contraindicated in women with one or more previous low transverse cesarean deliveries.
II. **Requirements for induction**
   A. Labor should be induced only after the mother and fetus have been examined and fetal maturity has been assured.
   B. **Criteria for fetal maturity**
      1. An ultrasound measurement of the crown-rump length, obtained at 6-11 weeks, supports a gestational age of 39 weeks or more.

2. An ultrasound obtained at 12-20 weeks, confirms the gestational age of 39 weeks or more determined by history and physical examination.
3. Fetal heart tones have been documented for 30 weeks by Doppler.
4. 36 weeks have elapsed since a positive serum or urine pregnancy test was performed.

C. If one or more of these criteria are not met, amniocentesis should be performed to document fetal maturity.

D. A cervical examination should be performed immediately before cervical ripening or oxytocin (Pitocin) infusion.

III. Cervical ripening

A. In a significant proportion of postdate pregnancies, the condition of the cervix is unfavorable, and cervical ripening is necessary.

B. **Prostaglandin E2**

1. Prostaglandin E2 vaginal gel may be prepared and administered for cervical ripening as 5 mg in 10 cc gel intravaginally q4h.
2. Prostaglandin E2 gel is available in a 2.5-mL syringe which contains 0.5 mg of dinoprostone (Prepidil).
3. A prostaglandin vaginal insert (Cervidil, 10 mg of dinoprostone) provides a lower rate of release of medication (0.3 mg/h) than the gel. The vaginal insert has an advantage over the gel because it can be removed should hyperstimulation occur.
4. There is no difference in efficacy between vaginal or cervical routes. The vaginal route is much more comfortable for the patient.
5. The prostaglandin-induced cervical ripening process often induces labor that is similar to that of spontaneous labor. Prostaglandin E2 may enhance sensitivity to oxytocin (Pitocin).
6. Before initiating prostaglandin E2, a reassuring fetal heart rate tracing should be present, and there should be an the absence of regular uterine contractions (every 5 minutes or less). After prostaglandin E2 intravaginal gel is placed, the patient is continuously monitored for 2 hours, then discharged.
7. **Protocol for administration**
   a. The patient should remain recumbent for at least 30 minutes.
   b. Effects of prostaglandin E2 may be exaggerated with oxytocin (Pitocin); therefore, oxytocin induction should be delayed for 6-12 hours. If the patient continues to have uterine activity as a result of the prostaglandin E2 gel, oxytocin should be deferred or used in low doses.
   c. If there is insufficient cervical change with minimal uterine activity with one dose of prostaglandin E2, a second dose of prostaglandin E2 may be given 6-12 hours later.
8. **Side effects of prostaglandin E2**
   a. The rate of uterine hyperstimulation is 1% for the intracervical gel, usually beginning within 1 hour after the gel is applied. Pulling on the tail of the net surrounding the vaginal insert will usually reverse this effect.
   b. Terbutaline, 250 mg SC or IV will rapidly stop hyperstimulation.

IV. Amniotomy.
Artificial rupture of membranes results in a reduction in the duration of labor. Before and after amniotomy the cervix should be palpated for the presence of an umbilical cord, and the fetal heart rate should be assessed and monitored.

V. Oxytocin (Pitocin)

A. Oxytocin administration stimulates uterine activity. No physiologic difference between oxytocin-stimulated labor and natural labor has been found.

B. **Administration**

1. Oxytocin is diluted 10 units in 1 liter (10 mU/ mL) of normal saline solution. Starting dosage is 0.5-2 mU/min, with increases of 1-2 mU/min increments, every 30-60 minutes.
2. A cervical dilation rate of 1 cm/h in the active phase indicates that labor is progressing sufficiently.

C. Side effects
  1. **Uterine hyperstimulation**
     a. The most common adverse effect of hyperstimulation is fetal heart rate deceleration. Decreasing the oxytocin dose rather than stopping it may correct the abnormal pattern. Uterine hyperstimulation or a resting tone above 20 mm Hg between contractions can lead to fetal hypoxia.
     b. Additional measures may include changing the patient to the lateral decubitus position, administering oxygen, or increasing intravenous fluid. When restarting the oxytocin, the dose should be lowered.
  2. Oxytocin does not cross the placenta; therefore, it has no direct effects on the fetus.
  3. Hypotension is seen only with rapid intravenous injection of oxytocin.

References: See page 140.

Postpartum Hemorrhage

Obstetric hemorrhage remains a leading causes of maternal mortality. Postpartum hemorrhage is defined as the loss of more than 500 mL of blood following delivery. However, the average blood loss in an uncomplicated vaginal delivery is about 500 mL, with 5% losing more than 1,000 mL.

I. Clinical evaluation of postpartum hemorrhage
  A. **Uterine atony** is the most common cause of postpartum hemorrhage. Conditions associated with uterine atony include an overdistended uterus (eg, polyhydramnios, multiple gestation), rapid or prolonged labor, macrosomia, high parity, and chorioamnionitis.
  B. **Conditions associated with bleeding from trauma** include forceps delivery, macrosomia, precipitous labor and delivery, and episiotomy.
  C. **Conditions associated with bleeding from coagulopathy and thrombocytopenia** include abruptio placentae, amniotic fluid embolism, preeclampsia, coagulation disorders, autoimmune thrombocytopenia, and anticoagulants.
  D. **Uterine rupture** is associated with previous uterine surgery, internal podalic version, breech extraction, multiple gestation, and abnormal fetal presentation. High parity is a risk factor for both uterine atony and rupture.
  E. **Uterine inversion** is detected by abdominal vaginal examination, which will reveal a uterus with an unusual shape after delivery.

II. Management of postpartum hemorrhage
  A. **Following delivery** of the placenta, the uterus should be palpated to determine whether atony is present. If atony is present, vigorous fundal massage should be administered. If bleeding continues despite uterine massage, it can often be controlled with bimanual uterine compression.
  B. **Genital tract lacerations** should be suspected in patients who have a firm uterus, but who continue to bleed. The cervix and vagina should be inspected to rule out lacerations. If no laceration is found but bleeding is still profuse, the uterus should be manually examined to exclude rupture.
  C. **The placenta and uterus should be examined** for retained placental fragments. Placenta accreta is usually manifest by failure of spontaneous placental separation.
  D. **Bleeding from non-genital areas** (venous puncture sites) suggests coagulopathy. Laboratory tests that confirm coagulopathy include INR, partial thromboplastin time, platelet count, fibrinogen, fibrin split products, and a clot retraction test.
  E. **Medical management of postpartum hemorrhage**
     1. **Oxytocin (Pitocin)** is usually given routinely immediately after delivery to stimulate uterine firmness and diminish blood loss. 20 units of oxytocin in 1,000 mL of normal saline or Ringer's lactate is administered at 100 drops/minute. Oxytocin should not be given as a rapid bolus injection because of the potential for circulatory collapse.
     2. If uterine massage and oxytocin are not effective in correcting uterine

atony, methylergonovine (Methergine) 0.2 mg can be given IM, provided there is no hypertension. If hypertension is present, 15-methyl prostaglandin F2-alpha (Hemabate), one ampule (0.25 mg), can be given IM, with repeat injections every 20min, up to 4 doses; it is contraindicated in asthma.

Treatment of Postpartum Hemorrhage Secondary to Uterine Atony	
Drug	**Protocol**
Oxytocin	20 U in 1,000 mL of lactated Ringer's as IV infusion
Methylergonovine (Methergine)	0.2 mg IM
Prostaglandin (15 methyl PGF2-alpha [Prostin/15M])	0.25 mg as IM every 15-60 minutes as necessary

F. **Volume replacement**
1. Patients with postpartum hemorrhage that is refractory to medical therapy require a second large-bore IV catheter. If the patient has had a major blood group determination and has a negative indirect Coombs test, type-specific blood may be given without waiting for a complete cross-match. Lactated Ringer's solution or normal saline is generously infused until blood can be replaced. Replacement consists of 3 mL of crystalloid solution per 1 mL of blood lost.
2. A Foley catheter is placed, and urine output is maintained at greater than 30 mL/h.

G. **Surgical management of postpartum hemorrhage.** If medical therapy fails, ligation of the uterine or uteroovarian artery, infundibulopelvic vessels, or hypogastric arteries, or hysterectomy may be indicated.

H. **Management of uterine inversion**
1. The inverted uterus should be immediately repositioned vaginally. Blood and/or fluids should be administered. If the placenta is still attached, it should not be removed until the uterus has been repositioned.
2. Uterine relaxation can be achieved with a halogenated anesthetic agent. Terbutaline is also useful for relaxing the uterus.
3. Following successful uterine repositioning and placental separation, oxytocin (Pitocin) is given to contract the uterus.

References: See page 140.

Uterine Infection

I. **Pathophysiology**
A. The major predisposing clinical factor for pelvic infections is cesarean delivery The frequency and severity of infection are greater after abdominal delivery than after vaginal delivery. The incidence of infection after vaginal delivery is only 1-3%, whereas the incidence after abdominal delivery is 5-10 times greater. Those patients who undergo elective cesarean section (with no labor and no rupture of membranes) have lower infection rates than do those who undergo emergency or nonelective procedures (with labor, rupture of membranes, or both).
B. Prolonged labor and premature ruptured membranes are the two most common risk factors associated with infection after cesarean birth. The number of vaginal examinations, socioeconomic status, and internal fetal monitoring have also been implicated.
C. Endometritis is a polymicrobial infection, with a mixture of aerobes and

anaerobes. Aerobes include gram-negative bacilli (eg, E coli) and gram-positive cocci (eg, group B streptococci). Anaerobic organisms have major roles in infection after cesarean birth; they are found in 80% of specimens. The most common isolated organism is Bacteroides.

II. Clinical evaluation

A. The diagnosis of endometritis is based on the presence of fever and the absence of other causes of fever. Uterine tenderness, especially parametrial, and purulent or foul-smelling lochia are common.

B. Laboratory studies, with the exception of blood cultures, are usually not helpful.

III. Treatment

A. Clindamycin-gentamicin most effective regimen, a combination that is curative in 85-95% of patients.

    a. Gentamicin 100 mg (2 mg/kg) IV load, then 100 mg (1.5 mg/kg) IV q8h.

    b. Clindamycin, 600-900 mg IV q8h.

B. Treatment with ampicillin (2 gm IV q4-6h) and an aminoglycoside is less effective in postcesarean endometritis. Good results have been reported with cefoxitin (1-2 gm IV q6h), cefoperazone (1-2 gm IV/IM q8h), cefotaxime, piperacillin, and cefotetan. Antibiotics containing a penicillin derivative and a beta-lactamase inhibitor are also effective.

C. Treatment is continued until the patient has been afebrile for 24-48 hours. Further antibiotic therapy on an outpatient basis is generally not necessary.

D. Causes of initial failure of antibiotic therapy include the presence of an abscess, resistant organisms, a wound infection, infection at other sites, or septic thrombophlebitis. Surgical drainage, especially for an abscess, may occasionally be necessary, although hysterectomy is rarely required.

References: See page 140.

Postpartum Fever Workup

History: Postpartum fever is ≥ 100.4 F (38 degrees C) on 2 occasions >6h apart after the first postpartum day (during the first 10 days postpartum), or ≥101 on the first postpartum day. Dysuria, abdominal pain, distention, breast pain, calf pain.

Predisposing Factors: Cesarean section, prolonged labor, premature rupture of membranes, internal monitors, multiple vaginal exams, meconium, manual placenta extraction, anemia, poor nutrition.

Physical Examination: Temperature, throat, chest, lung exams; breasts, abdomen. Costovertebral angle tenderness, uterine tenderness, phlebitis, calf tenderness; wound exam. Speculum exam.

Differential Diagnosis: UTI, upper respiratory infection, atelectasis, pneumonia, wound infection, mastitis, episiotomy abscess; uterine infection, deep vein thrombosis, pyelonephritis, pelvic abscess.

Labs: CBC, SMA7, blood C&S x 2, catheter UA, C&S. Endometrial Pipelle sample or swab for gram stain, C&S; gonococcus, chlamydia; wound C&S, CXR.

References

References may be obtained at www.ccspublishing.com/ccs

Index